CORONARY ARTERIAL VARIATIONS IN THE NORMAL HEART AND IN CONGENITAL HEART DISEASE

CORONARY ARTERIAL VARIATIONS IN THE NORMAL HEART AND IN CONGENITAL HEART DISEASE

ZEEV VLODAVER, M.D.

Senior Research Associate in Cardiovascular
Pathology, Miller Division–United Hospitals, St. Paul and
Research Associate, Graduate School,
University of Minnesota, Minneapolis, Minnesota

HENRY N. NEUFELD, M.D.

Chief, Heart Institute, Chaim Sheba Medical Center, Tel-Hashomer
and Professor of Medicine and Chaim Sheba Professor of Cardiology,
Sackler School of Medicine, Tel Aviv University, Tel Aviv, Israel

JESSE E. EDWARDS, M.D.

Director of Laboratories, Miller Division–United Hospitals, St. Paul and
Professor of Pathology, Graduate School,
University of Minnesota, Minneapolis, Minnesota

ACADEMIC PRESS, Inc.

New York   San Francisco   London   1975

A Subsidiary of Harcourt Brace Jovanovich, Publishers

Preparation for publication by
THE ISRAEL JOURNAL OF MEDICAL SCIENCES, Jerusalem

ACADEMIC PRESS, INC.
111 Fifth Avenue, New York, New York 10003

United Kingdom Edition published by
ACADEMIC PRESS, INC. (LONDON) LTD.
24/28 Oval Road, London NW1

Supported in part by
The National Library of Medicine
Public Health Service
U. S. Department of Health, Education, and Welfare
Bethesda, Maryland

Library of Congress Cataloging in Publication Data

Vlodaver, Zeev.
   Coronary arterial variations in the normal heart
and in congenital heart disease.

      Bibliography: p.
      Includes index.
      1.   Heart—Abnormalities and deformities.
2.   Heart—Anatomy.   3.   Coronary arteries—Abnormalities and deformities.   I.   Neufeld, Henry N.,
joint author.   II.   Edwards, Jesse E., joint author.
III.   Title.   [DNLM: 1.   Coronary vessels anomilies.
2.   Coronary vessels.   3.   Heart defects, congenital.
WG300 V871c]
RC687.V58   616.1'23'043   73-2086
ISBN 0–12–722450–5

CONTENTS

CONTENTS

PREFACE

This monograph contains the results of research on the coronary artery in infants and children. It is, we believe, the first presentation of a comprehensive study in which all aspects of the subject are considered—including prenatal and postnatal findings, and the differences between ethnic groups. The variation of origin of the coronary arteries and the differences in coronary patterns in congenital heart abnormalities are outlined in detail, as is the effect of a number of metabolic diseases on the coronary arteries.

As a result of these findings, a number of points relevant to the overall study of coronary heart disease have become evident. The seeds for coronary heart disease may be present even in the embryo, with possible differences in various ethnic groups. This difference may be expressed as an alteration of the norm in the coronary arteries or as a genetic factor predisposing to coronary arteriosclerosis.

It is our hope that this study, which throws additional light on the etiology and natural history of the development of coronary heart disease, will help the pediatrician, the cardiologist, the radiologist and the epidemiologist in their clinical work and research in coronary heart disease.

This book is another demonstration of the bridge that exists between the United States and Israel. The roots for this work were established in Israel and grew in the United States with the final work achieved through joint efforts of the authors from both continents.

H. N. NEUFELD

CHAPTER I

SINGLE CORONARY ARTERY

Single coronary artery is a rare anomaly that has to be considered even without other cardiac malformations as a pathologic entity. Without any additional malformations, cardiac function is normal and compatible with normal life expectancy in the majority of cases. There seems to be, however, an extra hazard when an individual with single coronary artery develops atherosclerotic changes in this artery which might cause problems of coronary disease to be noted clinically.

DEFINITION AND CLASSIFICATION

The definition of single coronary artery is as follows: 1) only one ostium is present; 2) the coronary artery originating from the one ostium supplies the entire heart.

The most acceptable classification today is that of Smith (13) who

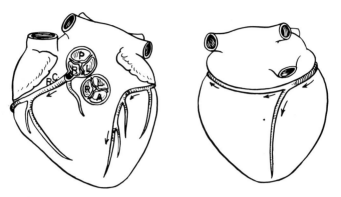

FIG. 1. Single coronary artery. The artery follows the course of one artery, in this instance, the right coronary artery (R.C.). P = posterior; R = right; L = Left; A = anterior aortic cusps. Same abbreviations are used in subsequent illustrations unless otherwise stated.

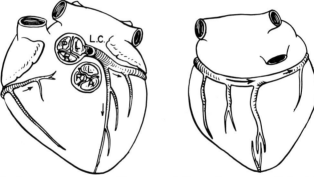

FIG. 2. Single coronary artery. The artery follows the course of the left coronary artery (L.C.).

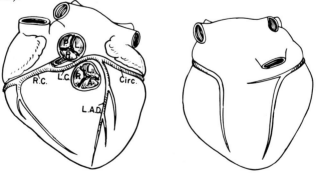

FIG. 3. Single coronary artery originating from right aortic sinus and then dividing into the right and left coronary arteries. Circ. = circumflex coronary artery; L.A.D. = anterior descending artery.

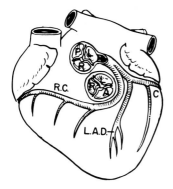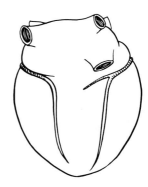

FIG. 4.   Single coronary artery arising from left aortic sinus and then dividing into right and left coronary arteries. The right artery runs anterior to the pulmonary trunk. C = circumflex coronary artery.

recognized three different types of single coronary artery as follows: Type I is a single coronary artery that follows the course of only one coronary artery, either the right (Fig. 1) or the left (Fig. 2). Type II is a single coronary artery that covers the distribution of two coronary arteries; in this type a single coronary artery arises from one ostium but divides in such a way that branches are present in the distribution of both right and left coronary arteries (Fig. 3 and 4). Smith (13) expressed the opinion that this type results from a misplaced anlage of a coronary artery which fuses in the initial portion of the normally arising anlage. Type III is a single coronary artery with so atypical a distribution that it cannot be compared with the normal pattern of either right or left coronary artery. We have encountered this situation only in association with other congenital cardiac malformations.

EMBRYOLOGY

As seen in the rabbit, the first anlage of the future coronary artery is a club-shaped bud which makes its appearance from the arterial surface of the bulbus arteriosus about the 12th day of embryonic life before the common trunk has been divided by the truncus septum into the aorta and pulmonary artery. The anlage of the left coronary artery appears somewhat later. Fish and amphibia have only one coronary artery, and only 60% of birds have two vessels. Mammals, however, generally have two coronary arteries. The development of two coronary arteries seems to be a late acquisition in evolution.

Roberts and Loube (11) proposed three possible mechanisms for the embryogenesis of this anomaly: 1) absence of the anlage of one coronary artery; 2) displacement of the anlage of one coronary artery so that it fuses with the anlage of the other; 3) closure of one coronary artery soon after its formation.

In the past, the presence of a single coronary artery was usually first identified at autopsy. With the increasing use of aortography, however, more cases diagnosed clinically are being reported.

No Other Congenital Cardiac Malformations

No intrinsic anomalies of the artery

Such a single coronary artery may originate as either a normal left or right coronary artery and 1) may continue to follow the normal course of that artery or 2) may branch into two main vessels, one of which follows approximately the normal course of the right coronary artery and the other that of the left coronary artery.

A single coronary artery was first reported by Hyrtl (8) in 1841, when he described a single left coronary artery in a fetus of seven months' gestation. Altogether about 150 cases have been found in the literature. In some of the case reports the clinical histories were inadequately described, and the details of the vascular patterns were only superficially outlined.

The sex ratio of males to females is 1.4:1.0 as reported by Allen and Snider (1) in a review of 69 cases. The incidence of single left or single right coronary artery seems to be equal. Patterns of distal distribution appear to be more variable for the single right coronary artery than for the single left coronary artery. The ages at which single coronary arteries have been observed range from the seven-month-old fetus described by Hyrtl (8) to 83 years as in the case reported by Causing and associates (3). Single coronary artery may appear with or without intrinsic abnormalities of the artery and with or without other cardiac anomalies. It is, however, found more commonly in conjunction with serious congenital cardiac defects than as an isolated condition.

With regard to single coronary artery without other cardiac malformations and without other intrinsic anomalies of the coronary arterial system, several authors have stated that myocardial ischemia may be expected. This would be especially pertinent when the single coronary artery is distributed primarily in the pattern of only one artery (1, 13). Most authors, however, have stressed that the condition is benign.

Davis (5) reported the case of a 50-year-old man whose electrocardiogram at the age of 34 years had shown signs of severe ischemia and probable myocardial infarction. The patient was asymptomatic, and despite recommendations to the contrary, continued all activity. He died of acute myocardial infarction following exercise. Autopsy revealed a single coronary artery with a saddle plaque occluding one of the branches of the artery.

We know of two examples (4, 7) in which a single coronary artery was identified during life. In one of these cases autopsy was performed and confirmed the presence of a single coronary artery. One of these cases, reported by Chapman and Peterson (4), was that of a 24-year-old man in whom an electrocardiogram revealed myocardial infarction in the diaphragmatic aspect of the left ventricle. Arteriography revealed a single left coronary artery arising from the anterior descending artery. Halperin and associates (7) reported the case of a 27-year-old woman who presented with congestive heart failure during pregnancy. Coronary arteriography revealed a single left coronary artery. Five months later she was readmitted to the hospital because of dyspnea. Nine days later, ventricular tachycardia developed, and the patient died. Autopsy confirmed the presence of a single (left) coronary artery. No atherosclerosis, thrombosis, or occlusion of the coronary arterial system was found.

It has been claimed that the single coronary artery is probably more prone to atherosclerosis than are the two normally arising coronary arteries. In single coronary artery, the consequences of arteriosclerosis may be particularly serious, since collaterals from a second coronary artery are not present, Thus, occlusion of the proximal portion of a single coronary artery would carry a severe prognosis.

Intrinsic anomalies of the artery

A single coronary artery in the absence of other cardiac anomalies may show intrinsic anomalies such as aneurysm or abnormal communication.

Aneurysm. An aneurysm or aneurysmal dilatation is extremely rare in a single coronary artery. Only two instances have been described (3, 11). Whether the aneurysmal dilatation in these cases is congenital or acquired is not known. Causing and associates (3) reported this situation in an 83-year-old man in whom death was caused by rupture of the aneurysm resulting in cardiac tamponade. This patient had only one coronary ostium that lay in the left aortic sinus. The artery divided into left circumflex and anterior descending branches while there was no evidence

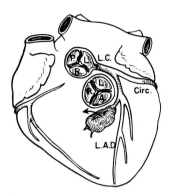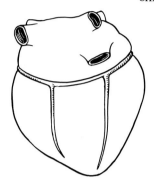

FIG. 5.   Single coronary artery arising from the left aortic sinus. The vessel branches into anterior descending and left circumflex vessels; the latter, which continues into the right atrioventricular sulcus, supplies the distribution of the right coronary artery. In this instance, a saccular aneurysm of a branch of the anterior descending coronary artery was present and had ruptured. (Modified from ref. 3.)

of a right coronary artery. Three and one-half centimeters from its bifurcation, the left anterior descending branch gave a branch to the right ventricle. This branch showed localized aneurysmal dilatation. The left circumflex branch coursed in the left atrioventricular groove and ultimately supplied the right ventricle (Fig. 5).

Anomalous communication. The coexistence of a single coronary artery and anomalous communication of the artery with a cardiac chamber or vein is an extremely rare condition and only a few cases have been described in the literature (6, 9).

Murray (10) reported on two patients, each with a single coronary artery which communicated with the right ventricle. In one of his patients, recovery followed ligation of the anomalous communication. The anatomic features in Murray's surgically treated patient are shown in Fig. 6. In this case, a single coronary artery arose from the usual site of the left coronary artery. A right branch arose 2.5 cm from the origin of the single coronary artery. It traversed the right atrioventricular groove and had the usual distribution and branching of a right coronary artery. Proximal to the origin of the posterior descending artery, the right branch exhibited a wide communication with the right ventricle.

Ruddock (12) and Anselmi and associates (2) described two similar cases; in each of these treatment was surgical. Michaud and co-workers (9) described three patients with coronary artery-right ventricular communication, one of whom had a single left coronary artery.

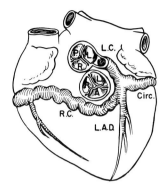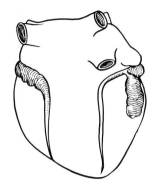

FIG. 6. Single coronary artery arising from the left aortic sinus and branching into right and left coronary arteries. Anomalous communication of the right coronary artery with the right ventricle accounts for enlargement of the main stem and the right and circumflex branches. (Modified from ref. 10.)

Hallman and associates (6), with the use of angiography, identified a single ("left") coronary artery, the posterior descending branch of which communicated with the right ventricle. In addition to ligating the anomalous communication of the single coronary artery to the right ventricle, Hallman and associates placed a Dacron graft between the aorta and the right ventricular portion of the coronary artery to establish dual coronary supply. The latter was done to protect against the hazard of atherosclerotic occlusive lesions in later life.

In those rare conditions in which a single coronary artery communicates with one of the ventricular chambers, the hemodynamics are similar to the condition in which one of two coronary arteries makes an anomalous communication with one of the cardiac chambers. When the communication is with the right atrium, right ventricle, or pulmonary artery, a left-to-right shunt exists. When the communication is with the left side of the heart, a condition simulating aortic insufficiency would be expected.

OTHER CONGENITAL CARDIAC MALFORMATIONS

Single coronary artery may be associated with other congenital cardiac malformations. In those instances, the distribution of the vessel is usually atypical. Among the 45 cases of single coronary artery reviewed by Smith (13), 15 belonged to this category. The coexistence of a single coronary artery with other congenital malformations of the heart seems to be more frequent than single coronary artery alone. No comprehensive review on this subject is available at present. On the following pages, we shall

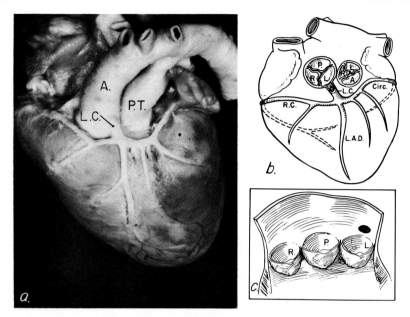

FIG. 7. Single coronary artery in a case of complete transposition of the great vessels. *a.* The single coronary artery (L.C.) arises from the left aortic sinus. The vessel then branches into right (R.C.) and left (L.C.) coronary arteries A. = aorta; P.T. = pulmonary trunk. *b.* Diagrammatic portrayal of the condition present as seen from the exterior. *c.* Opened aorta showing the ostium of the single coronary artery in relation to left aortic sinus (L.).

present examples of this condition which we have encountered in both the United Hospitals—Miller Division, St. Paul, Minnesota, and the Heart Institute of the Chaim Sheba Medical Center, Tel Hashomer, Israel.

This subject is also covered in Chapter IX, which deals with patterns of distribution of coronary arteries in various congenital anomalies.

Complete transposition of great vessels

The patient was a one-month-old girl who had been cyanotic since birth. A murmur was discovered two days after birth and congestive cardiac failure developed at that time. She was digitalized and referred to the hospital for further investigation. Angiocardiography demonstrated complete transposition of the great vessels, associated with patent ductus arteriosus; the presence of patent foramen ovale was also established. Signs and symptoms of failure continued in spite of intensive medical therapy and the child died at the age of one month.

Postmortem examination revealed complete transposition of the great vessels, patent ductus arteriosus, patent foramen ovale and a single coronary artery which arose above the left anterior aortic sinus. The artery divided into three branches: the right coronary was small and ran anterior to the aorta, the left circumflex was positioned anteriorly to the pulmonary trunk and the anterior descending artery followed a normal path (Fig. 7).

Origin of both great vessels from right ventricle

A single coronary artery was observed in association with origin of both great vessels from the right ventricle in a 23-month-old cyanotic female infant in whom a clinical diagnosis of asplenia had been made. This diagnosis was based in part upon the finding of Howell-Jolly bodies in the peripheral blood smear and an asymptomatic liver. The pathologic findings, in addition to confirming the diagnosis of asplenia, revealed a series of intracardiac malformations commonly seen in the asplenic syndrome. These included a common atrioventricular valve, a stenotic bicuspid pulmonary valve, a right aortic arch, persistent left superior vena cava joining the left atrium, absence of the coronary sinus and total anomalous pulmonary venous connection to the right superior vena cava. The aorta, which was wider than the pulmonary trunk, arose to the right of the latter and exclusively from the right ventricle. The pulmonary trunk also arose from the right ventricle.

The single coronary artery arose from the right posterior aortic sinus

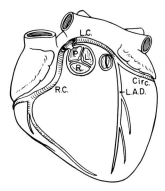

FIG. 8. Single coronary artery in a case of origin of both great vessels from the right ventricle with subpulmonary stenosis. The single coronary artery originates from the posterior aortic sinus and immediately branches into right and left coronary arteries.

and immediately divided into two branches. One of these pursued the course of a left coronary artery and, in turn, gave rise to the anterior descending and circumflex branches, while the other continued in the course of the right coronary artery (Fig. 8).

Pulmonary atresia with intact ventricular septum and hypoplastic right ventricle

The subject was a five-day-old, full-term, cyanotic female infant. Autopsy revealed pulmonary valvular atresia with intact ventricular septum, a large dilated right atrium and a patent ductus arteriosus. The ostium of the single coronary artery was less than 1 mm in diameter and originated from the left aortic sinus (Fig. 9). The artery branched into the anterior descending and left circumflex arteries. The latter vessel coursed in the left atrioventricular (AV) sulcus, continued posteriorly into the right AV sulcus and terminated along the anterior aspect of the right ventricle. Two posterior descending branches arose from this vessel posteriorly.

Persistent truncus arteriosus

A two-month-old infant was admitted to the hospital because of signs of congestive heart failure and upper respiratory infection. Cardiac catheterization revealed a persistent truncus arteriosus. The infant manifested severe, progressive cardiovascular failure. At autopsy, persistent truncus arteriosus, Type II, was found. Four semilunar cusps, left, right, anterior and posterior, were present; three of these were of equal size, whereas

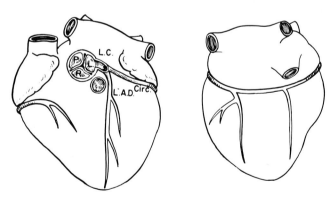

FIG. 9. Single coronary artery in a case of pulmonary valvular atresia with intact ventricular septum. This artery arises from the left aortic sinus and branches into anterior descending and circumflex vessels. The latter supplies the distribution of the right coronary artery.

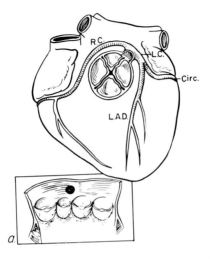

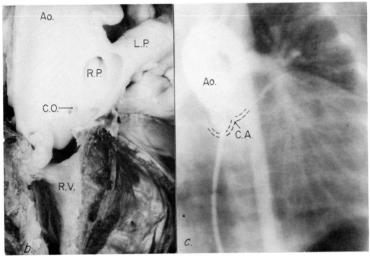

FIG. 10.   Single coronary artery in a case of persistent truncus arteriosus. *a.* Diagrammatic portrayal showing the single coronary artery arising at a high level above a commissure of a quadricuspid truncal valve. Shortly after its origin, the single vessel branches into right and left coronary arteries. Inset shows the position of the ostium of the single coronary artery. *b.* The specimen shows the interior of the truncus arteriosus from which the aorta (Ao.) and right and left pulmonary arteries (R.P. and L.P., respectively) arise. A ventricular septal defect is present immediately beneath the truncus valve. The single coronary artery (C.O.) arises above a commissure of a quadricuspid valve. R.V. = septal wall of the right ventricle. *c.* Aortogram showing the major vessels, as well as the origin of the single coronary artery (C.A.).

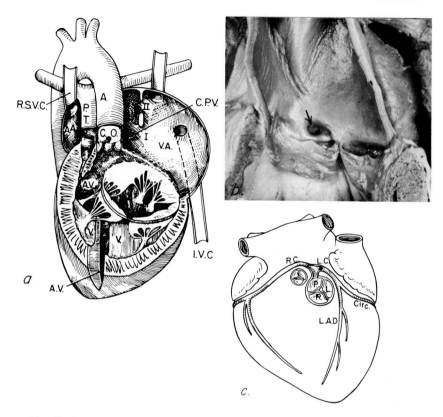

FIG. 11. Single coronary artery in a case of situs inversus with corrected transposition of great vessels and subpulmonary stenosis. *a.* Details of intracardiac malformations. A single coronary artery (C.O.) arises from the aorta. A.A. and V.A. = arterial atrium and venous atrium, respectively; V.V. = venous ventricle; R.S.V.C. = right superior vena cava. *b.* Interior of aorta showing ostium of single coronary artery (arrow). *c.* Distribution of the single coronary artery. The vessel arises from the posterior aortic sinus and bifurcates into right and left coronary arteries.

the posterior one was smaller. Above the commissure between the posterior and left cusps, a single 2-mm ostium was present from which a short coronary artery arose. The artery then bifurcated into vessels having the general course of the left and right coronary arteries (Fig. 10).

Origin of both great vessels from arterial ventricle in situs inversus
An additional example of a single coronary artery in association with congenital heart disease was seen in a seven-month-old female infant with

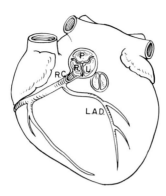

FIG. 12. Single coronary artery in a case of tetralogy of Fallot. The single coronary artery arises from the right aortic sinus and continues as a right coronary artery. The anterior descending coronary artery arises from the right coronary artery and crosses the infundibulum of the right ventricle to reach the anterior interventricular sulcus.

total situs inversus and bilateral superior venae cavae. Each superior vena cava joined the homolateral atrium. A common AV valve lay above a ventricular septal defect and led into the two ventricles which were of unequal size. The larger ventricle was on the right side and had the anatomic structure of a right ventricle. The smaller ventricle was on the left side and had the anatomic structure of a left ventricle (Fig. 11a). Each great artery arose from the right-sided ventricle, with the aortic valve lying to the left of the pulmonary valve. The three cusps of the aortic valve were oriented in right, left and posterior positions. The single coronary artery arose from the posterior aortic sinus (Fig. 11b). Shortly after its origin it divided into the right and left coronary arteries (Fig. 11c).

Tetralogy of Fallot

At the age of 11 years, the patient, a boy, underwent corrective surgery for tetralogy of Fallot. Fourteen months later, reoperation was performed because of a residual ventricular septal defect. At that time extensive adhesive pericarditis was present and a major coronary artery which crossed the outflow tract of the right ventricle was divided. After death, pathologic examination showed only one coronary ostium. This arose from the right aortic sinus. While the vessel pursued a course in the right AV sulcus, it gave off an anterior descending branch. That vessel crossed the right ventricular infundibulum as it proceeded to the anterior interventricular sulcus (Fig. 12).

One of us (H.N.N.) has observed a 13-year-old girl with tetralogy of Fallot in whom absence of the anterior descending branch of the left coronary artery was discovered at the time of surgery. This patient presented an intermittent electrocardiographic pattern of right ventricular hypertrophy alternating with a normal QRS pattern. Because of this finding we raised the question as to whether conduction disturbances might not play a greater role in the production of ventricular hypertrophy patterns than in tetralogy of Fallot with normal coronary arterial distribution and whether conduction disturbances might not be influenced by anomalous coronary flow.

REFERENCES

1. ALLEN GL and SNIDER TH. Myocardial infarction with a single coronary artery. Report of a case. *Arch Intern Med* **117**: 261, 1966.
2. ANSELMI G, MUNOZ S, BLANCO P, CARBONELL L and PUIGBO JJ. Anomalous coronary artery connecting with the right ventricle, associated with pulmonary stenosis and atrial septal defect. *Am Heart J* **62**: 406, 1961.
3. CAUSING WC, SHUSTER M and PRIBOR HC. Single coronary artery with ruptured coronary artery aneurysm. Report of a case. *Arch Pathol* **83**: 419, 1967.
4. CHAPMAN DW and PETERSON PK. Unusual forms of coronary disease as demonstrated by percutaneous coronary arteriography. *Med Rec (Houston)* **57**: 320, 1964.
5. DAVIS PL. Congenital absence of the left coronary artery. *Med Times* **90**: 293, 1962.
6. HALLMAN GL, COOLEY DA, McNAMARA DG and LATSON JR. Single left coronary artery with fistula to right ventricle. Reconstruction of two-coronary system with Dacron graft. *Circulation* **32**: 293, 1965.
7. HALPERIN IC, PENNY JL and KENNEDY RJ. Single coronary artery. Antemortem diagnosis in a patient with congestive heart failure. *Am J Cardiol* **19**: 424, 1967.
8. HYRTL J. Einige in chirurgischer Hinsicht wichtige Gefässvarietäten. *Med Jahrb Österreich St (Vienna)* **33**: 17, 1841.
9. MICHAUD P, FROMENT R, VIARD H, GRAVIER J and VERNEY RN. Coronaryright ventricular fistulas. Apropos of 3 operated cases. *Arch Mal Coeur* **56**: 143, 1963.
10. MURRAY RH. Single coronary artery with fistulous communication: report of two cases. *Circulation* **28**: 437, 1963.
11. ROBERTS JT and LOUBE SD. Congenital single coronary artery in man: report of nine new cases, one having thrombosis with right ventricular and atrial (auricular) infarction. *Am Heart J* **34**: 188, 1947.
12. RUDDOCK JC. Anomalous origin of left coronary artery. Case report. *US Nav Med Bull* **41**: 175, 1943.
13. SMITH JC. Review of single coronary artery with report of two cases. *Circulation* **1**: 1168, 1950.

CHAPTER II

VARIATION IN NUMBER OF
CORONARY OSTIA

Conus artery
Independent origins of left circumflex and anterior descending branches
Combinations of patterns

Otherwise normal or diseased hearts may vary from the classical pattern of two coronary arterial ostia in the aorta. Variations include the presence of a third (conus) artery and separate ostia for the anterior descending and circumflex arteries (Fig. 13).

CONUS ARTERY

Supernumerary coronary arteries have been observed since the days of the early anatomists. Little attention, however, has been given to them in most modern anatomy textbooks, and they are usually considered an uncommon variation and of little significance (2). Spalteholz (13) did not refer directly to this variation in his monograph. Grant (7) stated that "the accessory coronary arteries spring from the aortic sinus" in only 4% of hearts. There is no reference to supernumerary coronary arteries in Abbott's discussion of anomalies of the coronary arterial tree (1). In 1904, however, Banchi (3) injected a standard chalk mass into 100 hearts through the aorta and reported that the first ventricular branch of the right coronary artery arose directly from the sinus of Valsalva in 33% of human hearts and that he had found two such accessory arteries in 3% of hearts in his series. He called this accessory artery "adipose artery" and felt that it supplied the conus arteriosus and the superior portion of the sternocostal surface of the right ventricle. In 1910, Piquand (9) described his experience with the conus artery and stated that it was present in one-third of the hearts in human beings. Symmers (14), in 1907, determined the number of coronary arteries in 100 consecutive human

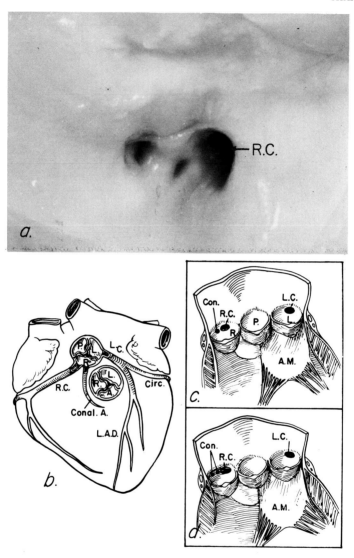

FIG. 13. Variations in the number of coronary ostia. *a*. Interior of aorta. Lying anterior to the ostium of the right coronary artery (R.C.) are two smaller ostia representing two conus arteries. *b*. A common situation in which a single conus artery arises anterior to the ostium of the right coronary artery as seen from the exterior of the heart. *c*. The situation portrayed in *b* viewed from inside the aorta. *d*. Two conus arteries (Con.) lie anterior to the right coronary artery, a feature similar to that shown in *a*.

hearts without regard to the presence of disease and found one or more accessory coronary arteries in 38% of cases. Classically, the diameters of these supernumerary vessels were small (0.5 to 2.0 mm), and they arose from the aorta anterior to and within a few millimeters of the mouth of the right coronary artery (Fig. 13). Crainicianu (5), in 1922, injected 200 hearts and found supernumerary vessels, which he called "alteria prae infundibularis," in 45% of his series. Chase and DeGaris (4) found 23 examples of accessory arteries in the coronary tree of 36 hearts of higher primates. Schlesinger and associates (11) referred to this type of accessory vessel as "the conus artery" and in studying 631 hearts found that, in 50% of their cases, the right infundibulum or conus was supplied by the conus artery which arose directly from the aorta. They were impressed by the fact that the conus artery often serves as a collateral vessel in the presence of obstructive coronary arterial disease. They also expressed the opinion that the amount of myocardial damage resulting from occlusion and narrowing of a coronary artery may be determined in part by the presence or absence of anastomoses between the conus artery and the rest of the coronary arterial tree.

INDEPENDENT ORIGINS OF LEFT CIRCUMFLEX AND ANTERIOR DESCENDING BRANCHES

Considerably less common than the presence of a conus arterial ostium in the aorta is the state in which there are separate aortic ostia for the anterior descending and left circumflex arteries. In this situation, the usual pattern is that both of the latter vessels arise from the left aortic sinus. Less commonly, the ostium of the left circumflex artery lies in the right aortic sinus posterior to the ostium of the right coronary artery.

Specific cases of separate origin of the left circumflex and left anterior descending branches from the left sinus (see Chapter IV, Fig. 27 and 28) were described in the literature (6, 8, 10, 12). James (8) found one case in 106 randomly selected hearts and Zumbo and associates (15), in a study of 2,089 consecutive autopsies, found separate origins of the two left branches in 21 cases (1%). A significantly lower incidence was observed by Schlesinger and associates (11). In studying 1,000 hearts, this group found four in which the left circumflex artery exhibited an independent origin. In two, this was from the left aortic sinus beside the ostium of the anterior descending artery. In the other two, the left circumflex arose from the right aortic sinus posterior to the origin of the right coronary artery.

The subject of independent origin of the left circumflex artery from the right aortic sinus will be considered further in a subsequent section.

COMBINATIONS OF PATTERNS

There are some cases in which more than three ostia are present (Fig. 13b and c). Usually, this pattern is a manifestation of the presence of more than one conus artery. Less commonly, independent origin of the left circumflex artery may yield three arteries arising from the aorta. This pattern of origin of the left circumflex artery may be associated with the presence of one or more conus arteries yielding four or more ostia in the aorta.

REFERENCES

1. ABBOTT M. Congenital cardiac disease, in Osler W and McCrae T (Eds), "Modern medicine," 3rd edn. Philadelphia, Lea and Febiger. 1927, v 4, chap 21, p 794.
2. ALEXANDER RW and GRIFFITH GC. Anomalies of the coronary arteries and their clinical significance. *Circulation* **14**: 800, 1956.
3. BANCHI A. Morfologia delle arteriae coronariae cordis. *Arch Ital Anat Embriol* **3**: 7, 1904.
4. CHASE RE and DeGARIS CF. Arteriae coronariae (cordis) in the higher primates. *Am J Phys Anthropol* **24**: 427, 1939.
5. CRAINICIANU A. Anatomische Studien über die Coronararterien und experimentelle Untersuchungen über ihre Durchlässigkeit. *Virchows Arch [Pathol Anat]* **228**: 1, 1922.
6. DEMANY MA and ZIMMERMAN HA. Congenital anomalies of the coronary arteries. A report of three cases. *Angiology* **18**: 370, 1967.
7. GRANT JCB. "A method of anatomy," 3rd edn. Baltimore, Williams and Wilkins, 1944.
8. JAMES TN. "Anatomy of the coronary arteries." New York, Paul B Hoeber, Inc, 1961.
9. PIQUAND G. Recherches sur l'anatomie des vaisseaux sanguins du coeur. *J Anat (Paris)* **46**: 310, 1910.
10. SCHILLHAMMER W. Fatal myocardial infarction in a young man with anomalous coronary arteries with terminal ventricular tachycardia. *Am Heart J* **46**: 613, 1953.
11. SCHLESINGER MJ, ZOLL PM and WESSLER S. The conus artery: A third coronary artery. *Am Heart J* **38**: 823, 1949.
12. SMOL'IANNIKOV A and NADDACHINA A. Anomalies of the coronary arteries. *Arkh Patol* **25**: 3, 1963.
13. SPALTEHOLZ W. "Die Arterien der Herzwand." Leipzig, S Hirzel, 1924.
14. SYMMERS WS. Note on accessory coronary arteries. *J Anat Physiol* **41**: 141, 1907.
15. ZUMBO O, FANI K, JARMOLYCH J and DAOUD AS. Coronary atherosclerosis and myocardial infarction in hearts with anomalous coronary arteries. *Lab Invest* **14**: 571, 1965.

CHAPTER III

POSITIONS OF CORONARY OSTIA

Spectrum of the normal
Ectopic positions

The ascending aorta may be divided into sinus and tubular portions; the sinus portion lies more proximally and is wider than the tubular portion. The junction between these two parts lies at about the level of the free edges of the aortic cusps.

SPECTRUM OF THE NORMAL

The levels of origin of the coronary arteries with respect to the junctional zone between the two parts of the ascending aorta vary considerably. Slight deviations in position from the junctional line may be termed "variations" from normal, whereas whenever a coronary artery arises above the junctional line by as much as 1 cm, the position may be termed an "ectopic position" or "high takeoff."

Little has been published regarding the variations in position of the coronary ostia. Banchi (2), in 1904, reported that the left coronary artery arose at the level of the free margin of the cusp in 48% of the cases, above the cusp margin in 34%, and below it in 18%. The right coronary artery arose at the level of the free margin of the cusps in 71% of the cases, above it in 19%, and below it in 10%.

In a study of 50 consecutive unselected adult hearts, we recognized four patterns of position of coronary ostia in the aorta (Fig. 14). The most common type (56% of the cases) was that in which both coronary ostia were positioned under the junctional line of the tubular and sinus parts of the aorta (Fig. 14a). In 30% of the cases, the right ostium was positioned below and the left ostium above the junctional line of the tubular and sinus parts of the aorta (Fig. 14b). In 8% of the cases the right ostium was above the junctional line and the left ostium below it (Fig. 14c), while in 6%, both coronary ostia were positioned above the line (Fig. 14d).

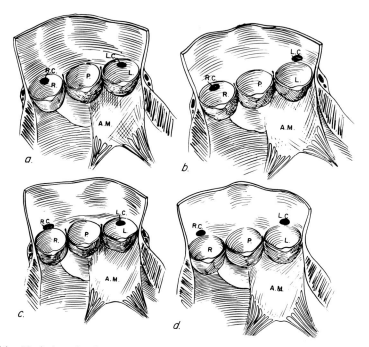

FIG. 14. Variations in the levels of origin of the coronary arteries. *a.* A common situation in which both the right (R.C.) and the left (L.C.) coronary arteries arise beneath the sinotubular junction of the ascending aorta. This anatomic arrangement was seen in 56% of cases. *b.* A situation seen in 30% of cases, in which the left coronary artery arises above and the right below the sinotubular junction of the aorta. *c.* In 8% of cases studied, the right coronary artery arose above the sinotubular junction and the left arose below it. *d.* In 6% of cases, both coronary arteries arose above the sinotubular junction of the aorta. A.M. = anterior leaflet of mitral valve.

ECTOPIC POSITION

With regard to ectopic or high takeoff positions of the coronary ostia, Gonzalez-Angulo and associates (4) described four cases in which both coronary arteries arose above the cusp margins, three cases in which the right coronary artery arose above the cusp and one case in which the left coronary artery arose above them. The greatest departure from the level of the cusp in the cases studied by Gonzalez-Angulo's group was 15 mm above the free margin of the cusp (Fig. 15).

Alexander and Griffith (1), in a series of 54 coronary artery anomalies, both major and minor in degree, found two cases in which both coronary

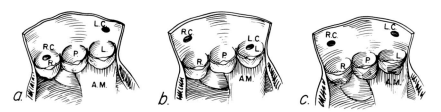

FIG. 15. Ectopic positions of origins of the coronary arteries with respect to the sinotubular junction of the aorta. *a.* The ostium of left coronary artery is excessively high. *b.* The ostium of the right coronary artery is excessively high. *c.* Both coronary arteries arise at excessively high levels from the tubular portion of the ascending aorta.

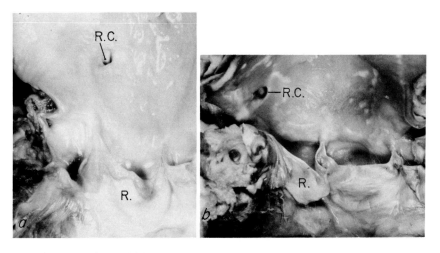

FIG. 16. Anomalously high origin of right coronary artery (R.C.) as seen in two specimens, *a* and *b.*

arteries arose above the aortic cusps, five in which only the right coronary artery arose high, and three in which only the left coronary artery was so involved.

Burck (3) reported two cases of high origin of the right coronary artery. He attributed the ischemia and death in one of these patients to the coronary lesion.

An example of an ectopic position is shown in Fig. 16.

REFERENCES

1. ALEXANDER RW and GRIFFITH GC. Anomalies of the coronary arteries and their clinical significance. *Circulation* **14**: 800, 1956.
2. BANCHI A. Cited in Blake HA, Manion WC, Mattingly TW and Baroldi G. Coronary artery anomalies. *Circulation* **30**: 927, 1964.
3. BURCK HC. Hoher und trichterförmiger Ursprung der Herzkranzarterien. *Beitr Pathol Anat* **128**: 139, 1963.
4. GONZALEZ-ANGULO A, REYES HA and WALLACE SA. Anomalies of the origin of coronary arteries. Special reference to single coronary artery. *Angiology* **17**: 96, 1966.

CHAPTER IV

PATTERNS OF ORIGIN OF CORONARY ARTERIES

Origin of both coronary arteries in relation to left aortic sinus
(Type I)
Origin of both coronary arteries in relation to right aortic sinus
(Type II)
Origin of left circumflex artery in relation to right aortic sinus
(Type III)
a) Independent of right coronary artery
b) From right coronary artery
Origin of anterior descending artery in relation to right aortic sinus
(Type IV)
a) Independent of right coronary artery
b) From right coronary artery
Origin of right coronary artery in relation to posterior
(noncoronary) aortic sinus (Type V.)
Independent origin of left circumflex and left anterior descending
arteries in relation to left aortic sinus (Type VI)

In hearts with normally related great vessels, with or without associated cardiac anomalies, the source of one or another coronary artery may be anomalous. Six types of patterns have been described or observed in our material (Fig. 17).

I. Origin of both coronary arteries in relation to left aortic sinus (Fig. 17a).

II. Origin of both coronary arteries in relation to right aortic sinus (Fig. 17b).

III. Origin of left circumflex artery in relation to right aortic sinus (Fig. 17c): a) independent of right coronary artery; b) from right coronary artery.

IV. Origin of anterior descending artery in relation to right aortic sinus (Fig. 17d): a) independent of right coronary artery; b) from right coronary artery.

[23]

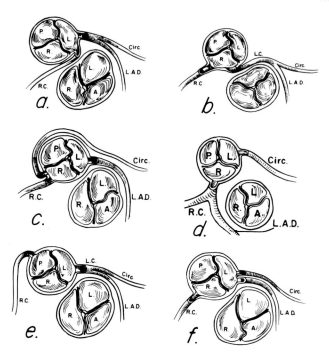

FIG. 17. Variation in pattern of origin of the coronary arteries. *a.* Type I: origin of both coronary arteries from left aortic sinus. *b.* Type II: origin of both coronary arteries from right aortic sinus. *c.* Type III: origin of the left circumflex coronary artery from the right aortic sinus posterior to normal site of origin of right coronary artery. *d.* Type IV: origin of anterior descending coronary artery from right coronary artery. *e.* Type V: origin of right coronary artery from posterior aortic sinus. *f.* Type VI: independent origin of left circumflex and anterior descending arteries from left aortic sinus. Same abbreviations as in Fig. 1–3.

V. Origin of right coronary artery in relation to posterior (noncoronary) aortic sinus (Fig. 17*e*).

VI. Independent origin of left circumflex artery and left anterior descending arteries in relation to left aortic sinus (Fig. 17*f*).

Origin of Both Coronary Arteries in Relation to Left Aortic Sinus (Type I; Fig. 17*a*)

The right coronary artery arises from the left aortic sinus anterior to the origin of the left coronary artery. The right artery runs between the

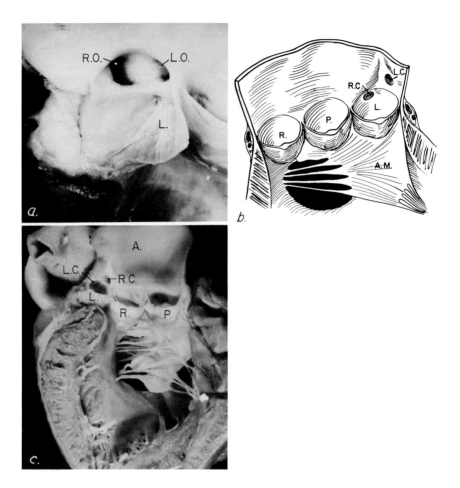

FIG. 18. Variations in origin of coronary arteries. *a.* In an otherwise normal heart, the right (R.O.) and left (L.O.) coronary ostia arise from the left aortic sinus. L. = retracted left aortic cusp. *b* and *c.* In a case of persistent common atrioventricular canal, both coronary arteries arise in relation to the left aortic sinus (L.). *b.* Diagram. *c.* The specimen.

ascending aorta and the pulmonary trunk to reach the right atrioventricular sulcus. The left coronary artery arises, courses and branches in the usual fashion (Fig. 18).

ORIGIN OF BOTH CORONARY ARTERIES IN RELATION TO RIGHT AORTIC
SINUS (TYPE II; FIG. 17*b*)

The situation wherein both the right and left coronary arteries originate from or above the right aortic sinus has been rarely reported. According to some authors, this anomalous condition may be a cause of sudden death in young persons and in adults (2). According to Benson, only four cases have been previously described (1, 3, 5). In the described cases, the left coronary artery originated in an oblique manner, very close to and anterior to the normal ostium of the right coronary artery. The left artery then passed between the great arterial trunks ultimately to achieve a normal position for the left coronary artery. The ages at death in the cases described by Benson and associates (1, 2) were between 11 and 14 years in three cases and 54 years in the fourth case.

In a case described by Cohen and Shaw (3), the patient, an 11-year-old boy, suffered an acute heart attack after running a short distance. He survived for 19 hours in the hospital, where clinical confirmation of myocardial infarction was obtained. Autopsy revealed that the left coronary artery arose immediately anterior to the right coronary ostium. It turned sharply toward the left, passed between the aorta and the pulmonary trunk, and branched as usual. The course of the main left coronary artery and the sharp angulation at its origin were believed to explain the coronary insufficiency and its fatal complication.

The first case described by Benson and Lack (2) was that of a 13-year-old boy who died suddenly after running. The origin and course of the left coronary artery were identical to those in the case described by Cohen and Shaw. Benson and Lack's second case was also that of a 13-year-old boy who died shortly after collapsing during a basketball game. In the 54-year-old patient described by Benson (1) in 1969, the left coronary artery showed much less atherosclerosis than the right. This observation led the author to speculate as to whether the left artery might have been subjected to less hemodynamic stress than the right coronary artery.

It is of interest that in all the cases described the patients were males and the left coronary artery was smaller than the right one. Therefore, one should be aware of this entity and recall it as a possible cause whenever sudden death occurs. This is probably especially indicated when males and younger persons die suddenly.

Origin of Left Circumflex Artery in Relation to Right Aortic Sinus (Type III; Fig. 19)

When the left circumflex artery arises from the right aortic sinus, two different subgroups may be recognized. In one, the left circumflex and right coronary arteries have independent ostia in the right aortic sinus

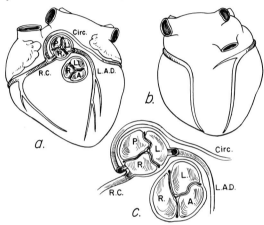

FIG. 19. Variation in origin of left circumflex coronary artery. *a* and *b*. A variation of the pattern of Type III in that the left circumflex coronary artery arises from the right coronary artery. *c*. The classical features of Type III as also shown in Fig. 17.

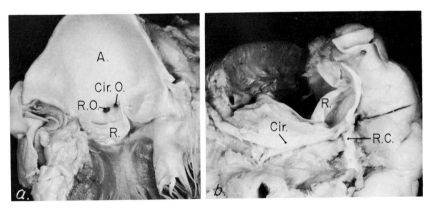

FIG. 20. Variation in origin of the coronary ostia, Type IIIa. *a*. The interior of the aorta (A.) shows the ostia of the right coronary (R.O.) and left circumflex (Cir. O.) arteries arising from the right aortic sinus. *b*. The right aortic sinus (R.) viewed from above, showing the origins of the left circumflex (Cir.) and right coronary (R.C.) arteries from this sinus.

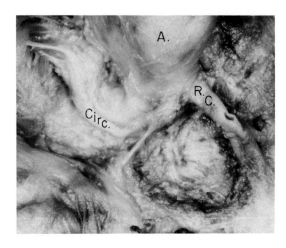

FIG. 21. Variation in origin of coronary artery, Type IIIa. In this example of congenital heart disease, which is characterized by supravalvular ring of the left atrium, ventricular septal defect and patent ductus arteriosus, the exterior of the aorta (A.) is viewed from behind, showing origins of the right (R.C.) and left circumflex (Circ.) coronary arteries in relation to each other. The left circumflex coronary artery crosses posteriorly to the aorta as it courses to the left atrioventricular sulcus.

(Fig. 20 and 21). In the second subgroup, the left circumflex coronary artery arises from the right coronary artery (Fig. 22–24). In both situations, the left circumflex artery courses posteriorly around the aorta and then runs inferior to the left atrial appendage to reach the left atrioventricular sulcus.

In both of the Type III patterns, the anterior descending coronary artery originates from the left aortic sinus at the usual site of origin of the main left coronary artery.

Origin of the left circumflex artery from the right aortic sinus is the most common type of abnormal pattern in coronary arterial origin and may be as frequent as one in 200 to 400 persons without other cardiac anomalies. In individuals with congenital heart disease, especially complete transposition, origin of the left circumflex artery from or in association with the right coronary artery is common.

This pattern of origin takes on a practical aspect with regard to coronary arterial perfusion during cardiac surgery. If only the left coronary artery is perfused, the myocardium in the distribution of the left circumflex artery is deprived. If only the right coronary artery is perfused, deficiency

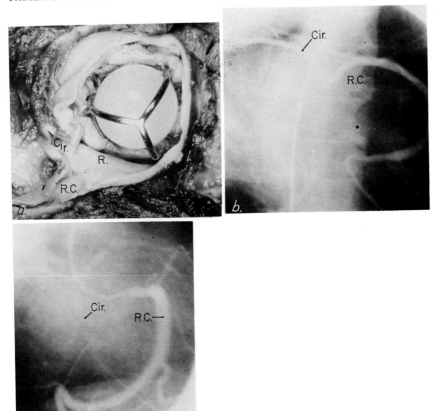

FIG. 22. Variation in origin of coronary arteries, Type IIIb. In a case of aortic valve replacement, the left circumflex coronary artery arose from the right coronary artery. *a.* The region of the aortic root, viewed from above, showing the aortic valvular prosthesis. Arising from the right aortic sinus (R.) is the right coronary artery (R.C.). The left circumflex coronary artery (Cir.) arises from the right coronary artery. During the operation, the right coronary artery was perfused beyond the origin of the left circumflex artery, leaving the distribution of the left ventricle in the distribution of the latter artery. *b* and *c.* Right coronary arteriograms showing the anomalous origin of the left circumflex coronary artery which circumflex coronary artery inadequately perfused, and resulting in necrosis of the left was illustrated in *a.* *b.* Frontal view. *c.* Right anterior oblique view.

in the distribution of the left circumflex artery may occur when the latter artery possesses an independent origin. If the circumflex artery arises from the right coronary artery near the aortic origin of the latter, the orifice of the perfusing cannula may lie beyond the site of origin of the

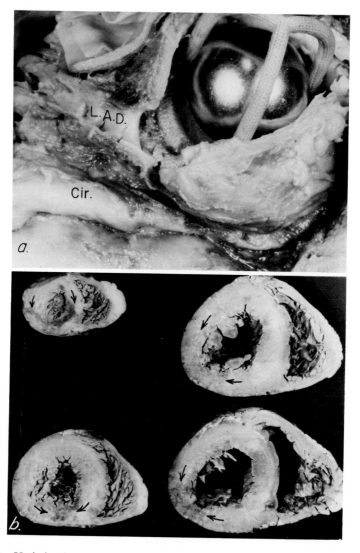

FIG. 23. Variation in origin of coronary arteries, Type IIIb. The situation is similar to that in Figure 22. *a.* View of aortic valvular prosthesis from above. The anterior descending coronary artery (L.A.D.) arises independently from the left aortic sinus. The left circumflex coronary artery (Cir.), which is shown entering the left atrioventricular sulcus, arose from the right coronary artery. After passing behind the aorta, it has reached the position shown in this illustration. *b.* Failure of perfusion of the left circumflex coronary artery during the replacement of the aortic valve resulted in infarction (between arrows) of the left ventricle in the distribution of this artery, as shown in cross sections of the left ventricle.

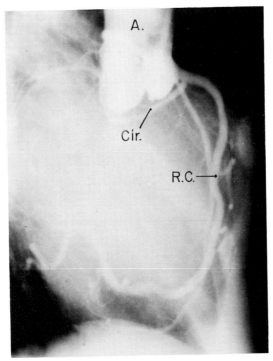

FIG. 24. Variation in origin of coronary arteries, Type IIIb. Lateral view of aortogram. The left circumflex coronary artery (Cir.) arises as a branch from the right coronary artery (R.C.). The anterior descending coronary artery can be seen in the background.

left circumflex, thus preventing perfusion of the myocardium which is supplied by the distribution of the latter artery (Fig. 22 and 23).

Lillehei and associates (6) described a case in which the left circumflex artery arose from the right coronary artery and perfusion was carried out only through the ostium of the left coronary artery during a surgical procedure. Following death of the patient, postmortem examination revealed signs of acute myocardial infarction in the distribution of the left circumflex coronary artery.

ORIGIN OF ANTERIOR DESCENDING ARTERY IN RELATION TO RIGHT AORTIC SINUS (TYPE IV; FIG. 25)

Anomalous origin of the anterior descending coronary artery is a variation of the coronary vasculature which is similar in some respects to

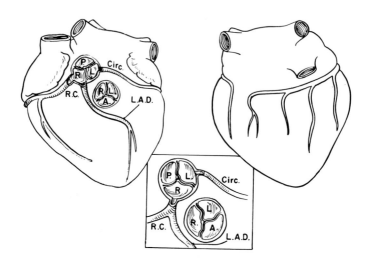

FIG. 25. Variation in origin of coronary arteries, Type IV. Two variations of this type are shown; each is characterized by the independent origin of the left circumflex coronary artery from the left aortic sinus, while the anterior descending coronary artery arises either from the right coronary artery (inset) or independently from the right aortic sinus.

origin of the left coronary artery from the right aortic sinus. Two circulatory patterns are recognized. In the first, the anterior descending coronary artery and the right coronary artery arise by separate ostia from the right aortic sinus. In the second pattern, the anterior descending coronary artery originates from the right coronary artery. In either case, the initial course of the anterior descending artery is similar to that of the conus artery. It then proceeds across the anterior aspect of the right ventricular infundibulum to reach the anterior interventricular sulcus. In each of the two foregoing patterns, the left circumflex artery arises independently from the left aortic sinus.

Meng and associates (7) described seven cases of tetralogy of Fallot in which the anterior descending coronary artery arose from the right aortic sinus; in four of the cases it was as a branch of the right coronary artery and in three it had an independent ostium.

In corrected transposition, the anterior descending artery arises from the right-sided coronary artery. In this situation, the pattern is part of the process of inversion which occurs in corrected transposition. With this view in mind, the anterior descending artery may be said to arise from an inverted anatomic left coronary artery.

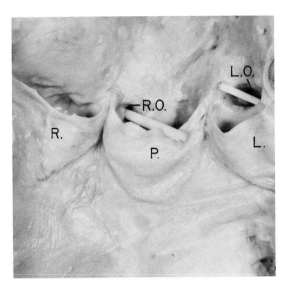

FIG. 26. Variation in origin of the coronary arteries, Type V. Origin of the right coronary artery (R.O.) from the posterior aortic sinus (P.). Left coronary artery (L.O.) arises normally from the left aortic sinus (L.) in the heart without congenital anomalies R. and L. = right and left aortic sinuses.

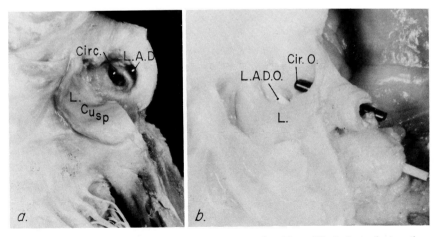

FIG. 27. Variation in origin of the coronary arteries, Type VI. Independent ostia of anterior descending (L.A.D.) and left circumflex (Circ.) coronary arteries from the left aortic sinus in two hearts each without congenital anomalies. a. The two ostia lie close together. b. The two ostia (L.A.D.O. and Cir. O.) are more separated from each other than those shown in a.

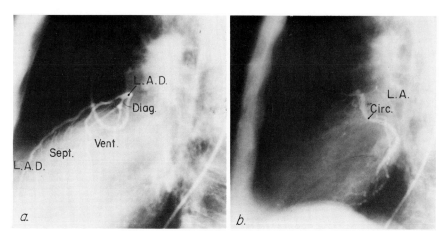

FIG. 28. Selective arteriograms showing variation in origin of coronary arteries, Type VI. Conditions shown in Fig. 27. *a.* The anterior descending coronary artery. L.A.D. = anterior descending artery; Diag. = diagonal branch; Sept. = septal branches; Vent. = ventricular branches. *b.* Left circumflex coronary artery. Circ. = left circumflex coronary artery; L.A. = left atrial branch.

ORIGIN OF RIGHT CORONARY ARTERY IN RELATION TO POSTERIOR (NONCORONARY) AORTIC SINUS (TYPE V; FIG. 26)

We have seen one example of this situation in a 72-year-old male with hypertension and coronary cardiovascular disease. The right coronary artery curves around the right aspect of the ascending aorta to reach the right atrioventricular sulcus. Although this pattern is uncommon or rare in association with a normally developed heart, it is common in complete transposition.

INDEPENDENT ORIGIN OF LEFT CIRCUMFLEX AND LEFT ANTERIOR DESCENDING ARTERIES IN RELATION TO LEFT AORTIC SINUS (TYPE VI; FIG. 27 AND 28)

This subject has been considered in the section dealing with variations in the number of coronary ostia. From independent origins, the anterior descending and left circumflex arteries proceed to their usual territories of distribution (4, 8).

REFERENCES

1. BENSON PA. Anomalous aortic origin of coronary artery with sudden death: Case report and review. *Am Heart J* **79**: 254, 1969.

2. BENSON PA and LACK AR. Anomalous aortic origin of left coronary artery. *Arch Pathol* **86**: 214, 1968.
3. COHEN LS and SHAW LD. Fatal myocardial infarction in an 11-year-old boy associated with a unique coronary artery anomaly. *Am J Cardiol* **19**: 420, 1967.
4. JAMES TN. "Anatomy of the coronary arteries." New York, Paul B Hoeber, Inc, 1961.
5. JOKL E, McCLELLAN JT and ROSS GD. Congenital anomaly of left coronary artery in young athlete. *JAMA* **182**: 572, 1962.
6. LILLEHEI CW, BONNABEAU RC JR and LEVY MJ. Surgical correction of aortic and mitral valve disease by total valve replacement. *Geriatrics* **19**: 240, 1964.
7. MENG CC, ECKNER FA and LEV M. Coronary artery distribution in tetralogy of Fallot. *Arch Surg* **90**: 363, 1965.
8. ZUMBO O, FANI K, JARMOLYCH J and DAOUD AS. Coronary atherosclerosis and myocardial infarction in hearts with anomalous coronary arteries. *Lab Invest* **14**: 571, 1965.

CHAPTER V

HYPOPLASTIC OR SHORT CORONARY ARTERIES

Hypoplasia of one coronary artery
Short left coronary artery

HYPOPLASIA OF ONE CORONARY ARTERY

A uniform narrow state of a coronary artery on the basis of intrinsic structure of the vessel is termed "hypoplasia" of the artery; either the right or left coronary artery and their branches may be involved. This state may exist either alone or in conjunction with other cardiac anomalies (1) (Fig. 29).

When the left system is hypoplastic, the right coronary artery tends to be enlarged and gives off the posterior descending artery and also supplies a considerable extent of the lateral wall of the left ventricle. In contrast, when the right artery is hypoplastic, the posterior descending artery is derived from the left circumflex artery, while the right coronary artery tends to terminate shortly after its marginal branch is given off. Hypoplasia of a main coronary artery is compatible with long life; in most of the reported cases the patients are over 60 years of age. Nevertheless, sudden death has been reported, as in the 26-week-old patient of Wenger and Peace (3).

Kjaergaard (2) reported a case of a woman who died suddenly. She had presented a history of fainting spells from the age of 29 years. These

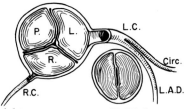

FIG. 29. Hypoplasia of right coronary artery (R.C.) in a case of tetralogy of Fallot.

[36]

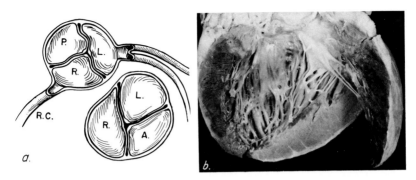

FIG. 30. Short left coronary artery. *a.* After a short course, the main left coronary artery bifurcates into its two usual branches. Cannulation during operation may result in perfusion either of the circumflex or of the anterior descending artery, while the other vessel is obstructed from a source of blood supply. *b.* Left ventricle. Acute necrosis of anteroseptal region following replacement of aortic valve. During the operation, cannulation of the left coronary artery appears to have resulted in cannulation of the left circumflex artery beyond a short left coronary artery, leaving the anterior descending vessel without perfusion. Death occurred one day after operation.

became more severe and she developed paroxysmal ventricular tachycardia and Adams-Stokes attacks prior to her death at the age of 39 years. Several members of this patient's family died from cardiac causes. At necropsy, a hypoplastic left circumflex branch was found together with left ventricular hypoplasia.

SHORT LEFT CORONARY ARTERY (FIG. 30*a*)

In adults, the left coronary artery normally runs about 9 to 12 mm before branching into its terminal branches, but it is not uncommon for it to be less than 1 cm long. The practical importance of this variation is that during cannulation the tip of the cannula may enter one of the branches, usually the anterior descending, and deprive the other branch of perfusion (Fig. 30*b*).

REFERENCES

1. ALEXANDER RW and GRIFFITH GC. Anomalies of the coronary arteries and their clinical significance. *Circulation* **14**: 800, 1956.
2. KJAERGAARD H. Coronary-arterial hypoplasia with paroxysmal tachycardia and sudden death. *Acta Med Scand* **135**: 439, 1949.
3. WENGER NK and PEACE RJ. Rudimentary left coronary artery. *Am J Cardiol* **8**: 519, 1961.

CHAPTER VI

CONGENITAL ANEURYSM OF A CORONARY ARTERY

Congenital aneurysm of a coronary artery is a very rare condition. Most coronary arterial aneurysms have some underlying lesion, such as atherosclerosis or an anomalous communication of a coronary artery with a cardiac chamber or the pulmonary trunk. Although localized aneurysms in the setting of an anomalous communication have been called "congenital" by some authorities, we prefer to consider them acquired complications of a congenital condition.

As used here, the term "congenital aneurysm" refers to a state in which the aneurysm is not associated with other congenital lesions of the coronary arterial system. The designation of an aneurysm as congenital implies only that the basic cause is developmental. The actual development of aneurysmal dilatation based on structural weakness may occur during the neonatal period but may not appear for decades. According to Packard and Wexler (7), the first report of an aneurysm of the coronary artery was made by Bougon in 1812 (2). In 1957, Crocker and associates (3) reviewed the literature and found 68 cases. Congenital deficiency involving the elastic elements of the media at the bifurcation of the vessels was originally suggested by Forbus (4) in 1930 as responsible for cerebral aneurysm and he further suggested that the same causative factor may operate in so-called congenital aneurysm of the coronary artery. Harris (5), in 1937, reported a case of "cirsoid aneurysm" of the right coronary artery; the underlying cause, he believed, was deficiency of elastic tissue. Ashton and Munro (1) described, in 1948, an unusual case of a 23-year-old male who died suddenly while playing football. Autopsy revealed, in addition to a loculated hydatid cyst of the liver, an aneurysm of the left coronary artery. About 1 cm from its origin, this artery showed localized dilatation and atheroma. Scott (8), in 1948, reviewed 47 cases of coronary artery aneurysms in the literature and considered that 15 of them

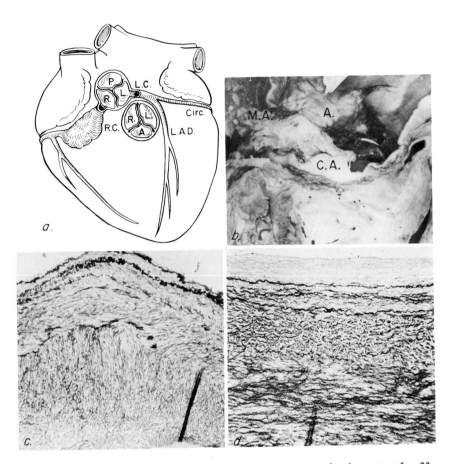

FIG. 31. Congenital aneurysm of the right coronary artery in the case of a 33-year-old patient with aortic insufficiency secondary to bacterial endocarditis of the aortic valve. *a*. Diagram. *b*. The anterior aspect of the ascending aorta (A.) has been removed, exposing a mycotic aneurysm of the aorta (M.A.). The proximal portion of the right coronary artery (C.A.) is aneurysmal. Histologic evidence indicates a congenital aneurysm as shown in *c* and *d*. *c*. Longitudinal section of aneurysm of the right coronary artery. No evidence of inflammatory reaction. The medial layer is thick and composed of an outer circular and an inner longitudinal smooth muscle layer. Elastic tissue stain; × 59. *d*. Transverse section of the aneurysm. Elastic tissue stain; × 44. From ref. 6.

were congenital. In 1968, Kalke and Edwards (6) described a congenital aneurysm of the proximal segment of the right coronary artery in a 33-year-old man with aortic insufficiency secondary to bacterial endocarditis of a

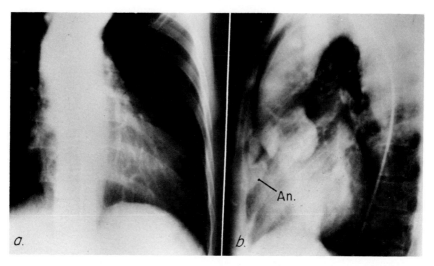

FIG. 32. Aortograms in the case of congenital aneurysm of the right coronary artery illustrated in Fig. 31. *a.* Frontal view. *b.* Lateral view. The aneurysm (An.) of the right coronary artery is more clearly shown in this perspective than in the frontal view. From ref. 6.

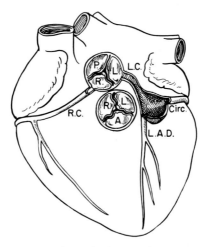

FIG. 33. Congenital aneurysm of terminal part of left coronary artery. Specimens from this case are shown in Fig. 34 and 35.

bicuspid aortic valve (Fig. 31). The artery did not show evidence of inflammatory disease. The coronary aneurysm had been noted in the preoperative aortogram (Fig. 32).

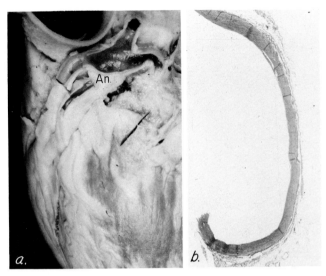

FIG. 34. Congenital aneurysm of terminal part of the left coronary artery. *a.* Left lateral view of the root of the aorta. The left coronary artery which divides into the anterior descending and left circumflex arteries shows an aneurysmal dilatation. *b.* Photomicrograph of the aneurysm. The wall is devoid of inflammatory or atherosclerotic disease. Elastic tissue stain; × 5.

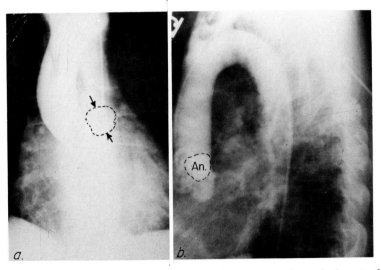

FIG. 35. Aortograms in the case of congenital aneurysm of terminal part of left coronary artery illustrated in Fig. 33 and 34. *a.* Frontal view. Opacification (between arrows) to the left of the root of the aorta caused by aneurysm. *b.* Lateral view. The shadow of the aneurysm (An.) lies within the dotted circle.

We observed the case of a 59-year-old man with chronic cor pulmonale and congestive heart failure in whom aortography had shown an aneurysm of the left coronary artery (Fig. 33–35). At necropsy, the terminal portion of the left coronary artery and proximal segment of the anterior descending coronary artery in continuity showed an aneurysm measuring 22 mm in length and 1.2 mm in width (Fig. 34a). Histologically, the media of the aneurysm showed a mosaic pattern in which elastic fibers intermingled with groups of smooth muscle cells (Fig. 34b). The intima was slightly thickened with nonspecific connective tissue. No atheromatous formation was present.

REFERENCES

1. Ashton H and Munro M.   Coronary artery aneurysm with occlusion due to a calcified thrombus. *Br Heart J* **10**: 165, 1948.
2. Bougon and Wexler *Bibl Med* **37**: 85, 1812, cited by Packard (7).
3. Crocker DW, Sobin S and Thomas WC.   Aneurysm of the coronary arteries. Report of three cases in infants and review of the literature. *Am J Pathol* **33**: 819, 1957.
4. Forbus WD.   On the origin of miliary aneurysms of the superficial cerebral arteries. *Bull Johns Hopkins Hosp* **47**: 239, 1930.
5. Harris PN.   Aneurysmal dilatation of the cardiac coronary arteries: Review of the literature and report of a case. *Am J Pathol* **13**: 89, 1937.
6. Kalke B and Edwards JE.   Localized aneurysms of the coronary arteries. *Angiology* **19**: 460, 1968.
7. Packard M and Wexler HF.   Aneurysm of the coronary arteries. *Arch Intern Med* **43**: 1, 1929.
8. Scott DH.   Aneurysms of the coronary arteries. *Am Heart J* **36**: 403, 1948.

CHAPTER VII

ANOMALOUS COMMUNICATION OF A CORONARY ARTERY WITH A CARDIAC CHAMBER OR MAJOR THORACIC VESSEL

DEFINITION

In the absence of intracardiac malformations, there are two major situations in which a coronary artery may communicate with a cardiac chamber or the pulmonary trunk.

In the first situation, both coronary arteries arise in normal fashion from the aorta, but a branch of a coronary artery connects directly with 1) one of the four cardiac chambers or the coronary sinus or superior vena cava or 2) the pulmonary trunk. When a branch of a coronary artery enters the pulmonary trunk directly, the presumption is that this vessel is an accessory coronary artery arising from the pulmonary trunk that connects with one or more branches of the normally arising coronary

[43]

arteries. Such vessels make collateral communication with the ramifications of one or both of the usual coronary arteries.

In the second situation, one coronary artery arises from the aorta and the contralateral one arises from the pulmonary trunk. This condition is referred to as anomalous origin of a coronary artery from the pulmonary trunk (1). This subject is dealt with separately in Chapter VIII.

Clinical recognition of communications of a coronary artery with a cardiac chamber or the pulmonary trunk, although an uncommon anomaly, is important for several reasons. Such a fistula enters into the differential diagnosis of conditions associated with a continuous precordial murmur. It may be a cause of congestive heart failure, bacterial endocarditis, or both. Furthermore, as has been shown by Björck and Björck (12), it may be treated surgically.

The incidence of coronary artery fistula in cases of congenital heart disease was 0.26% in the series reported by Gasul's group (38) and 0.40% in McNamara and Gross's series (60). From these figures, one would expect a population incidence of about one in 50,000. There does not appear to be any particular sex preference.

EMBRYOLOGY

In early prenatal life, the coronary arteries communicate with the veins through a classic capillary network. The arteries also give off branches to the intertrabecular spaces which, in turn, communicate with the ventricular cavities. In late prenatal life, the intertrabecular spaces shrink to form the sinusoids which represent communications between the veins and coronary arteries, on the one hand, and the cardiac chambers, on the other (42). Abnormally large connections of the type that later form communication of an artery with a cardiac chamber appear to represent persistence of the large intertrabecular spaces which connect with the ventricular cavity, on the one hand, and a coronary artery on the other.

The explanation for anomalous communication between a coronary artery and the pulmonary trunk is different. The anomalous communication may be considered an accessory artery which makes communication with branches of one or both normally arising coronary arteries. Since flow from the high pressure aortic area is carried into the low pressure pulmonary area, the communication enlarges.

CORONARY ARTERY OF ORIGIN AND SITE OF ANOMALOUS TERMINATION

Our review of the literature in 1961 (70) yielded 50 cases of anomalous communications of coronary arteries. The artery involved and the site of termination of the communication are listed in Table 1.

Sakakibara and associates (77, 93) reviewed 118 cases of anomalous termination of coronary arteries in 1966, and McNamara and Gross (60) reviewed 172 cases in 1969. These reviews make it apparent that fistulae originating from the right coronary artery are somewhat more common than those from the left coronary artery. In four of the cases reported by McNamara and Gross, both coronary arteries were involved and in six the fistula arose from a single coronary artery. The great majority (more than 90%) emptied into the lesser circulation, the right ventricle being the most frequent recipient, followed in order of frequency by the right atrium and the pulmonary artery. Only 23 fistulae terminated in the left side of the heart: 17 in the left atrium and six in the ventricle. In one of the cases reported by Neufeld and associates (70), three openings were found in the pulmonary trunk. Characteristically, the coronary

TABLE 1. *Coronary artery involved and site of termination in 50 cases collected from the literature[a]*

Coronary artery involved	Reference no.	Site of termination	Cases	
			No.	%
Right	18, 26, 30, 31, 35, 47, 48, 51, 58, 63, 70, 73, 78, 93	Right atrium or cardiac vein	14	28
Right	32, 43, 70, 78, 90	Right ventricle	8	16
Right	1, 5, 9, 15, 80, 94	Pulmonary trunk	6	12
Total right		All	28	56
Left	14, 23, 33, 70	Right atrium or cardiac vein	4	8
Left	4, 16, 22, 65, 66, 70, 82, 87	Right ventricle	8	16
Left	6, 11, 69, 70, 79	Pulmonary trunk	5	10
Left	25, 54, 64, 70	Left atrium	3	6
Left	13, 57	Left ventricle	2	4
Total left		All	22	44
Total left and right			50	100

[a] From ref. 70.

arteries that enter into anomalous communication with the cardiac chamber or the pulmonary trunk are obviously enlarged, being not only dilated but also elongated and tortuous. A localized saccular aneurysm is a frequent finding in the enlarged artery. Calcification may complicate the saccular aneurysms. The artery that communicates anomalously fails to show dilatation only on rare occasions (20, 33).

CLINICAL FEATURES

The natural history of this malformation is not well known. In most cases reported in the literature, the patients are asymptomatic and in those in which the surgical repair was undertaken, the indication for surgery was the prevention of the development of complications such as bacterial endocarditis and rupture of the fistula or a secondary saccular aneurysm. In those apparently rare instances in which the abnormal communication causes a large left-to-right shunt, symptoms may be present. These include palpitation, shortness of breath, recurrent respiratory infection and congestive heart failure, as observed in two of the six patients described by Neufeld and associates in 1961 (70).

In general, the clinical picture in coronary arteriovenous fistula presents a wide spectrum that ranges from no symptoms to those of severe congestive heart failure. Symptoms, when present, are usually secondary to congestive heart failure which, in turn, results from a large left-to-right shunt. In those patients in whom a coronary artery fistula is associated with other cardiac malformations, the clinical picture may be dependent upon the severity and type of the associated lesion. Symptoms tend to appear in two age groups, namely in early infancy (3, 19, 23, 24, 46, 49) and after the age of 40 years (3, 9, 11, 23, 24, 53, 69, 96). Atrial fibrillation is frequent in older patients with coronary artery fistulae and may precipitate congestive heart failure (12, 18, 23, 36, 96, 97). Bacterial endocarditis or bacterial infection of the fistula occurs in about 10% of patients with coronary artery fistula and may represent the first clue to the cardiac anomaly (32, 38, 61, 62, 70, 76, 77, 84, 87, 90, 91).

Though saccular aneurysms of the coronary artery are commonly associated with fistulae, rupture of aneurysms is rare (7, 44). Angina and myocardial ischemia may occur. A striking finding is a continuous murmur, usually superficial in character, that can be best heard along the left lower sternal border. A thrill is usually associated. The murmur has been frequently confused with that of patent ductus arteriosus. Because of its location, however, it resembles more closely the murmur heard in ventricular septal defect associated with aortic insufficiency. In the case of large shunts leading to a cardiac chamber or vessel other than the left ventricle, diastolic pressure is frequently low and pulse pressure is elevated.

The second sound at the pulmonary area may be accentuated. It is of interest that, in Scott's case (80), a murmur was absent. Perhaps this could be explained by the finding at necropsy of a thrombus occluding the fistula.

Phonocardiography has been used to substantiate the murmur in many cases. In some instances, intracardiac phonocardiography has been performed at the time of cardiac catheterization. This allowed precise localization of the termination of the fistula and confirmed that the continuous murmur arose at the site of the anomalous connection rather than along the involved artery (48). Some patients manifest symptoms and signs of coronary insufficiency as shown in one of our cases (70). In those cases in which the anomalous termination is into the left ventricle, only a diastolic murmur is anticipated. A continuous murmur, however, was also noted in McNamara and Gross's two cases of left ventricular communication (60).

The electrocardiogram is not specific and may show various abnormalities depending upon the anatomic situation and associated alteration in hemodynamics. If the left-to-right shunt is small, no specific abnormal findings will appear on the electrocardiogram. If, however, a large shunt exists, signs of left ventricular hypertrophy may be found. A large shunt was present in only one of our patients (70), and that patient's electrocardiogram revealed signs of left ventricular overwork. In those instances in which a coronary artery anomalously connects with the right atrium or a tributary vein, both left ventricular hypertrophy and right ventricular volume overload patterns may occur, as observed in the case reported by Edwards and associates (26). In the case of an 80-year-old man reported by Colbeck and Shaw (18) involving anomalous communication between the right coronary artery and the right atrium, the electrocardiogram showed atrial fibrillation and left bundle-branch block. At necropsy, the heart weighed 554 g; left ventricular hypertrophy and dilatation were noted. Evidence of right atrial hypertrophy may be associated occasionally with fistulae to the right atrium (95). In the great majority of reported cases in which atrial fibrillation occurs, the fistulae terminate in the right atrium or coronary sinus.

The roentgenogram is not diagnostic, although unusual cardiac silhouettes have been reported on the basis of aneurysmal dilatation of the involved coronary artery (12, 31, 39, 53, 80, 86, 93). In the majority of patients with fistulae to the right side of the heart, some increase in pulmonary vascularity is shown in the roentgenogram. In an occasional case, the fistulous vessel itself may be sufficiently large so that it creates one or several convexities along the border of the heart in which it lies. Such a pseudoaneurysmal appearance when associated with evidence of a left-to-right shunt should suggest the possibility of communication of a coronary artery with a cardiac chamber.

When a fistula is to the outflow tract of the right ventricle, its precise localization may be difficult angiographically. This results from the fact that the contrast material passes rapidly from the right ventricle to the pulmonary artery. Nevertheless, correlation with catheterization data will usually lead to the correct diagnosis.

HEMODYNAMICS

The important functional disturbance of this condition is abnormal runoff of blood from the coronary arterial system, a state similar to that in other arteriovenous fistulae. Consequently, when a coronary artery communicates with a chamber on the right side of the heart, cardiac catheterization may reveal elevated levels of oxygen in the blood in the chamber receiving the fistula. When an abnormal communication exists with the left side of the heart, no abnormality in oxygen saturation will be discovered at cardiac catheterization. In reports, calculated shunts—when the anomalous communication was with the right side of the heart— varied from minimal 0.6 to 8.7 liters/min per m² of body surface (70). Pressures in the pulmonary arteries and the right intracardiac chambers were, in most instances, within normal limits. Hemodynamic studies may readily permit the identification of the site of anomalous communication of a coronary artery with a right heart chamber or vessel. They do not, however, reveal the anatomic basis for the shunt. Precise anatomic diagnosis requires selective aortography which is the diagnostic method of choice in this condition.

The size and area of communication appear to be important factors in regulating blood flow through the communication. The larger the fistula, the greater wil be the volume of blood shunted. However, certain aspects regarding the size of fistula may become manifest during ventricular systole. A fistula to the right ventricle usually passes through the myocardium and, with contraction of the myocardium during systole, the communication is reduced and so is the amount of blood shunted. Such an obstruction may be sufficient to prevent flow completely during systole.

The site of the fistulous opening also influences the flow since it plays a role in regulating the pressure and resistance gradients. Flow to the right ventricle usually shows diastolic accentuation. This is because of the constriction of the fistula during systolic contraction. During diastole, the communication enlarges, there is less resistance to flow and the shunt increases over that during ventricular systole.

With time, flow through the involved coronary artery gradually increases. This leads to increased dilatation, length and tortuosity of the involved artery.

Hudspeth (50) described a case of an anomalous communication of the right coronary artery to the right atrium, in which pressures and flow values were measured directly at the time of operation. With the fistula intact, the pressure at the root of the aorta was 120 mm Hg and flow through the fistula was 737 ml/min leaving an effective myocardial blood flow of only 50 ml/min. After the fistula was resected, total flow in the right coronary artery was reduced to 122 ml/min. Nevertheless, this represented a trebling of the effective myocardial flow. After obliteration of the fistula, the pressure in the distal coronary artery was 100 mm Hg. According to Hudspeth (50), considerable interference with coronary arterial blood flow exists even with fistulae from a right coronary artery into the right side of the heart. Based on those observations, Hudspeth postulated that the coronary circulation is abnormal in any patient with a coronary arteriovenous fistula, and he considered this condition as providing further support for surgical treatment of these lesions even in the asymptomatic patient. Normal perfusion pressure and adequate effective coronary arterial blood flow may be expected after obliteration of this fistula.

Dedichen and associates (24) reported data from a case of right coronary artery-pulmonary vein fistula. They found a flow of 1,800 ml/min through the involved artery. The flow curve pattern differed from the normal. Instead of the markedly phasic flow, the flow was almost constant, with a slight increase during systole. After the fistula was closed, the flow in the right coronary artery was reduced to about 250 to 300 ml/min.

Björk and Björk (12) felt that the heart with a coronary arteriovenous fistula could compensate adequately for long periods of time, even with large left-to-right shunts. Decompensation and congestive heart failure eventually supervene, usually in persons over 40 years of age, as a direct effect of the shunt upon blood flow to the myocardium.

The fact that myocardial ischemia and infarction are infrequent complications that appear only in the older patients, however, suggests that flow to the myocardium is usually adequate. Collateral circulation from the uninvolved coronary artery is a contributing factor to the adequacy of flow. Ischemia in extremities distal to an arteriovenous fistula is well recognized. It is reasonable to assume, therefore, that a large coronary fistula would similarly drain blood away from the coronary circulation and would also be responsible for lowering the pressure gradient across the myocardial capillary bed. McNamara and Gross (60) described four cases in which electrocardiographic changes suggested myocardial ischemia (26, 55, 60, 76, 93). Although angina occurs, it is not frequent (2, 8, 21, 24, 28, 59, 60, 70).

In the differential diagnosis of fistulae involving the coronary arteries, several conditions are to be considered. These include ventricular septal defect associated with aortic insufficiency, patent ductus arteriosus (22), aorticopulmonary septal defect and ruptured aortic aneurysm.

SURGICAL TREATMENT

The first surgical procedure in anomalous communication of a coronary artery was reported by Björck and Crafoord in 1947 (11). Surgical experience in 49 cases was reviewed by Taber and associates (88) in 1967, and in 1969, 91 operative cases were reviewed by McNamara and Gross (60).

Indications for surgical intervention include 1) prevention of bacterial infection, 2) rupture of a complicating saccular aneurysm of the involved artery and 3) congestive heart failure (26, 70, 93). Bacterial endocarditis had developed in four of the 46 cases reviewed by Taber and associates (88) in which operations were performed (10, 19, 61, 84). Congestive heart failure is most likely to develop when a fistula involving the coronary system is asociated with an additional shunt such as a patent ductus arteriosus (14, 61).

A variety of surgical approaches for obliteration of the fistula have been employed. Björck and Crafoord (11), in 1947, first successfully closed a fistula by ligating the involved coronary artery. This method is essentially in use today when the ligature may be placed close to the termination of the fistula (Fig. 36). When, however, a long segment lies proximal

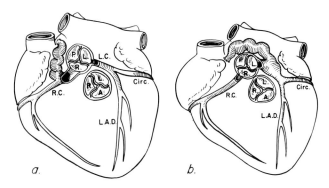

FIG. 36. Anomalous communication of coronary artery with lesser circulation. *a.* Right coronary artery communicates with right atrium. *b.* Left coronary artery communicates with right atrium.

to the fistula, it is common practice to ligate the involved branch at its arterial origin and at its termination. Experience has demonstrated that, with ligation of the involved coronary artery, myocardial ischemia is frequently observed (2, 3, 8, 11, 14, 24, 46, 78, 87), myocardial infarction is observed occasionally (8, 46, 61, 86) and ventricular fibrillation in some cases (46). Such experiences stress the importance of interruption of the anomalously connecting coronary artery beyond all branches which supply the myocardium.

The operative mortality associated with closure of a coronary artery fistula should be minimal, and in the 46 cases reviewed by Taber and associates (88), two postoperative deaths were reported. The deaths occurred in infants, five and 18 months of age, respectively. Each had had an untreated patent ductus arteriosus causing pulmonary hypertension and cardiomegaly (14, 61). In the 93 surgical cases reviewed by McNamara and Gross (60), a third death occurred. The patient, a 53-year-old woman, died from massive hemopericardium in the early postoperative period. To our knowledge, no other deaths have been reported after operations for uncomplicated coronary artery fistulae.

Kimbiris and associates (52), in 1970, reviewed 17 reported cases of anomalous communication of a coronary artery with the coronary sinus. To this number we added two from the literature (Table 2). Of 19 patients, eight underwent operations; no mortality occurred.

Among the reported surgical cases, the arteries involved and the sites of termination were essentially like those presented in the foregoing

TABLE 2. *Reported cases of coronary artery-coronary sinus or vein fistula*

Case no.	Age (years)/ sex	Ref. no.	Coronary artery involved		Reported symptoms	Murmurs	Electrocardiogram	X-rays	Diagnosis made by	Treatment
			R	Cir						
1	54 M	47	+	....	NR	Systolic	NR	NR	Autopsy	....
2	72 M	68	....	+	Precordial pain, palpitations, dizziness, dyspnea	NR	NR	NR	Autopsy	....
3	62 F	58	+	....	Heart failure for two years	NR	NR	NR	Autopsy	....
4	43 F	30	+	....	NR	NR	NR	NR	Autopsy	....
5	9 M	73	+	....	None	Continuous	Normal	NR	Thoracotomy for PDA	None
6	58 F	23	....	+	Heart failure	Continuous	AF	Cardiac enlargement, bilateral pleural effusion	Autopsy	....
7	8 F	94	?	?	None	Continuous	Normal	Increased pulmonary vascular markings, prominence of PA	Suspended by cardiac catherization	None

TABLE 2. (cont.)

Case no.	Age (years)/ sex	Ref. no.	Coronary artery involved		Reported symptoms	Murmurs	Electrocardiogram	X-rays	Diagnosis made by	Treatment
			R	Cir.						
8	4 F	78	+	...	General weakness, fatigue	Systolic and diastolic	LVH RBBB	RVH and LVH, increased pulmonary vascular markings, prominence of PA	Thoracotomy for ASD	Surgical ligation
9	12 F	2	...	+	Fatigue on exertion	Continuous	Normal	Prominence of PA	Thoracotomy for PDA	Surgical ligation
10	52 M	44	...	+	Chest pain	None	NR	NR	Autopsy	....
11	5 F	45	+	...	Cardiomegaly and upper respiratory infection	Continuous	LVH	Enlarged heart	Angiography	Operation
12	47 M	10	...	+	SBE	Systolic and early diastolic	Normal	Normal heart size, prominent hilar shadows	Thoracotomy for ASD	Surgical ligation
13	37 M	28	...	+	NR	NR	NR	NR	Selective coronary arteriography	Surgical ligation
14	13 F	21	+	...	Substernal pain on exertion, palpitations	Continuous	Mild LVH	Normal heart size, increased pulmonary vascular markings	Cineartography	Surgical ligation

TABLE 2. (*cont.*)

Case no.	Age (years)/ sex	Ref. no.	Coronary artery involved		Reported symptoms	Murmurs	Electrocardiogram	X-rays	Diagnosis made by	Treatment
			R	Cir.						
15	7 M	21	+	....	Substernal chest pain on strenuous exercise	Systolic and diastolic	LVH	Heart moderately enlarged, increased pulmonary vascular markings	Cineangiography	Surgical ligation
16	66 M	52	....	+	Heart failure, chest pain	Systolic and diastolic	1° AV block; nonspecific T wave changes	RVH, LVH, increased vascular markings	Catheterization angiography	
17	45 M	52	+	....	Heart failure, chest pain	Continuous	LVH	RVH, LVH, minimal increased pulmonary vascular markings	Cineangiography	
18	52 F	[a]	+	....	Heart failure, chest pain	Systolic and diastolic	Nonspecific T wave changes	RVH, LVH, minimal prominence of pulmonary vasculature	Catheterization and aortogram	Surgical ligation
19	23 days M	74	....	+	Heart failure	Systolic	—	—	Autopsy	

+ = involved; .... = not involved.
ASD = atrial septal defect; AV = atrioventicular; Cir = circumflex; LVH = left ventricular hypertrophy; NR = not reported; PA = pulmonary artery; PDA = patent ductus arteriosus; RVH = right ventricular hypertrophy; SBE = subacute bacterial endocarditis; RBBB = right bundle-branch block.

[a] Karnegis JN, Johnson T and Castaneda AR (unpublished data).

TABLE 3.   *Review of 93 operative cases with coronary artery fistula*[a]

Coronary artery origin	No. of cases	Site of termination	No. of cases	Reference no.
Right	55	Right ventricle	48	3, 20, 28, 34, 46, 61, 67, 70, 71, 75–78, 82, 85, 88
Left	30	Right atrium	23	7, 10, 11, 14, 19, 21, 28, 34, 39, 40, 53, 64, 70, 75, 76, 77, 79, 88
Both	2	Pulmonary artery	13	11, 12, 24, 28, 67, 70, 77
Single	6	Left atrium	7	8, 24, 28, 54, 64, 75, 81
		Left ventricle	2	60

[a] From ref. 60.

section dealing with pathology. The details relative to the operative cases are summarized in Table 3.

Isolated patients reported by Neill and Mounsey (69) and Sakakibara and associates (77) were found to have residual murmurs after operation. These were attributed to the reappearance of the fistula. Otherwise, most of the patients described in the literature remained asymptomatic after operation. Within one year, most patients showed a regression of cardiomegaly and a decrease of pulmonary vascular congestion, when these conditions had been present.

Communication with a Specific Chamber or Vessel
Right atrium (Fig. 36)

In 66 of the 200 cases of anomalous communication of a coronary artery with a cardiac chamber or a thoracic vessel reviewed by Oldham and associates (72), the anomalous termination was in the right atrium, coronary sinus, or the superior vena cava.* In the 42 surgically treated cases

---

* No distinction was made between the relative incidence of those three types of termination. Since we are aware of reports of anomalous communication of a coronary artery with the coronary sinus in 19 instances and with the superior vena cava in three instances, it is probable that the right atrium was the site of termination in about 44 of the cases reviewed by Oldham and associates.

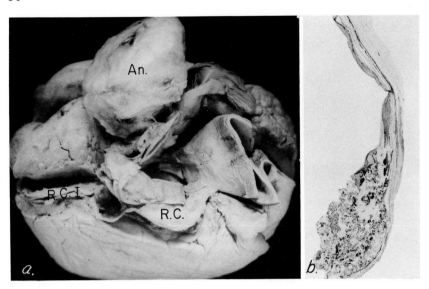

FIG. 37. Anomalous communication of the right coronary artery with the right atrium in a 53-year-old woman. *a.* The heart viewed from above. The right coronary artery (R.C.) is grossly dilated at its origin and gives rise to a branch which proceeds posteriorly. This dilated branch communicates with the cavity of the right atrium and, proximal to this, the communication shows an aneurysm (An.). The right coronary artery (R.C.I.) beyond the branch leading to the right atrium is of normal caliber. *b.* Photomicrograph of the wall of the saccular aneurysm. Residual medial tissue is present in the artery. In addition, there is a focus of intimal calcification. Elastic tissue stain; ×16. From ref. 26.

reviewed by Taber and associates (88), the anomalous communication was with the right atrium, coronary sinus, or superior vena cava in nine instances (12, 14, 36, 40, 64, 70, 76, 79).

When the right atrium is involved, the specific site to which the artery connects may be the anterior wall of the chamber or the region of the sinus node (Fig. 37).

In the review by Oldham et al. (72), the vessel involved was named in 62 of the 66 cases in which the anomalous communication terminated in the right atrium, coronary sinus or superior vena cava. The right, left, or both coronary arteries were involved in 41, 18 and three cases, respectively.

Coronary sinus (Fig. 38)

A fistula between a coronary artery and the coronary sinus is an un-

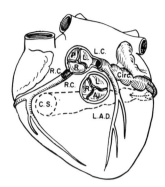

FIG. 38.   Anomalous communication of left circumflex coronary artery with coronary sinus (C.S.).

common anomaly. To our knowledge, only 19 cases have been reported (Table 2). Of these cases, seven were first diagnosed at autopsy (23, 30, 44, 47, 58, 68) and four during thoracotomy performed for a diagnosis other than this condition (2, 10, 73, 78). One was suspected after cardiac catheterization (94). Only seven were diagnosed preoperatively by angiocardiography (43, 45), selective arteriography, or both (28, 83).

The first case of coronary artery-coronary sinus fistula was reported by Halpert (47) in 1930. The patient, a 54-year-old man, died of cancer of the stomach. The fistula was a coincidental finding at autopsy. Several recent cases are reviewed below. Haller and Little (45), in 1963, reported the first case diagnosed by angiocardiography.

Haller and Little's patient, a five-year-old girl, was admitted to the hospital because of cardiomegaly and upper respiratory infection. Examination disclosed a moderately loud continuous murmur. No thrills were palpable. The murmur was best heard to the left of the sternum in the fourth and sixth intercostal spaces and extended toward the apex. The electrocardiogram revealed evidence of left ventricular hypertrophy. The thoracic roentgenogram showed a large heart with a contour that was suggestive of left ventricular enlargement. The pulmonary vasculature was within normal limits. By cardiac catheterization, a left-to-right shunt at the atrial level was detected; the ratio of pulmonary flow to systemic blood flow was 2.1 : 1. The pulmonary arterial pressure was 55 mm Hg systolic and 15 mm Hg diastolic with a mean of 28 mm Hg. No evidence of peripheral stenosis of the pulmonary artery could be demonstrated. Selective aortography demonstrated aneurysmal dilatation of the right

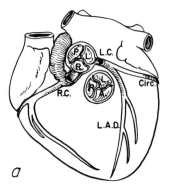
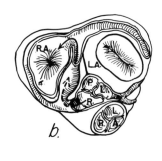

FIG. 39. Anomalous communication of right coronary artery with coronary sinus.
a. Frontal view.   *b.* View from above.

coronary artery with flow into the right atrium. The child was operated on, and before the pericardium was opened, a striking continuous thrill was palpable over the right atrium. The first 2 to 3 cm of the right coronary artery were markedly enlarged, but the distal branches were not unusual (Fig. 39). Through the posterior wall of the right atrium, the coronary sinus felt like a tense structure. Localized point pressure over the right coronary artery resulted in obliteration of the thrill. The fistula involved a branch of the right coronary artery which arose 0.5 cm distal to the aortic origin of the parent vessel. The fistula measured 1 cm in length and terminated in a greatly dilated tributary of the coronary sinus.

Effler and co-workers (28), in their series of 15 cases of abnormal communication of coronary arteries, found only one case of coronary artery-coronary sinus fistula. Croom and associates (21) recently reported two cases of right coronary artery-coronary sinus fistula diagnosed by aortography.

One of their patients was a seven-year-old boy, in whom cardiomegaly was discovered on routine physical examination. The child's development had been normal and he had been asymptomatic except for several episodes of substernal chest pain brought on by strenuous exertion. On examination, a grade II/VI (on a grading basis of I to VI) systolic ejection murmur was heard along the left sternal border and a grade II/VI diastolic murmur was heard over the left precordium. No precordial thrills were palpable. There was no evidence of congestive heart failure. The electrocardiogram revealed signs of left ventricular hypertrophy.

The thoracic roentgenogram showed moderate cardiomegaly with increased pulmonary vasculature. Right-heart catheterization showed normal pressures and an oxygen step-up of 1.5 vol. % was found in the right atrium. Selective aortography (cineangiography) revealed a large tortuous right coronary artery which appeared to lead to the right side of the heart. At the time of operation, a markedly dilated right coronary artery was found to arise from the aorta. The artery descended into the right atrioventricular groove and then turned acutely to enter the right atrium in the region of the coronary sinus ostium. In the latter location, a sharply localized continuous thrill was palpable.

The same authors described another patient, a 13-year-old girl, whose only complaints were occasional periods of substernal pain with strenuous exertion. Physical examination revealed a grade III systolic murmur, in addition to a continuous murmur of less intensity along the lower right sternal border. There was no evidence of congestive heart failure, and the electrocardiogram showed borderline left ventricular hypertrophy. The thoracic roentgenogram revealed some prominence of pulmonary arterial vasculature without cardiomegaly.

At operation, the right coronary artery arose from the aorta and was obviously dilated. It followed a very tortuous course in the right atrioventricular groove and then entered the heart in the region of the coronary sinus. The right coronary artery measured 3 cm in diameter at its origin. It then tapered gradually to a diameter of 0.5 cm at its entrance into the coronary sinus where a sharply localized continuous thrill was palpated. Each of the patients described by Croom and associates was successfully operated on.

Kimbiris and associates (52) described two cases. Their first patient, a 66-year-old woman, was admitted because of exertional dyspnea, easy fatigability, and frequent episodes of epigastric and thoracic pain associated with numbness of the left arm. A cardiac murmur had been discovered at age 36 and at age 48 the patient was treated for subacute bacterial endocarditis.

Physical examination revealed a grade III systolic ejection murmur at the second left intercostal space, and systolic and early diastolic murmurs were audible over the apex. Cardiac catheterization showed increased blood oxygen content at the right atrial level. Aortography demonstrated a normal ascending aorta and an extremely dilated and tortuous vessel that corresponded to the left circumflex coronary artery. Later, the coronary sinus, right atrium, right ventricle and pulmonary

artery were opacified. The anterior descending and the right coronary
arteries appeared normal.

The diagnosis of left circumflex coronary artery-coronary sinus fistula
was made, and the patient was operated upon. The findings at operation
confirmed the diagnosis. The fistula was interrupted surgically. The
patient did well postoperatively and the murmurs disappeared.

The second patient described by Kimbiris and associates (52), a 45-
year-old man, was admitted with complaints of substernal pressure-like
pain and exertional dyspnea of several months' duration. He was known
to have had a murmur for 25 years.

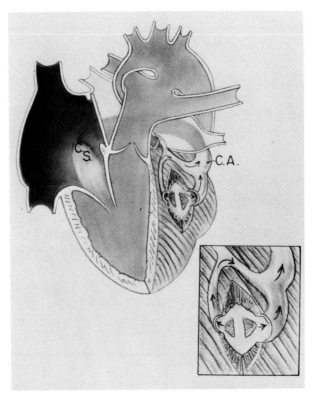

FIG. 40. Anomalous communication of left circumflex coronary artery with the
coronary sinus in a case of aortic atresia with premature closure of the foramen
ovale. The main body of the illustration shows the aortic atresia and the hypoplastic
left ventricle. Through sinusoids, the left ventricular cavity joins the left circumflex
coronary artery. The latter, in turn, joins the coronary sinus (C.S.). C.A. = left
circumflex coronary artery. Inset: Communications with cavity of left ventricle.
From ref. 74.

Physical examination revealed a continuous murmur over the third and fourth intercostal spaces just to the right of the sternum. An ejection click was heard at the left sternal border. The electrocardiogram revealed signs of left ventricular hypertrophy.

On cineaortography the ascending aorta and aortic valve appeared to be normal. The right coronary artery was extremely dilated and tortuous. Selective opacification of this right coronary artery demonstrated its communication with the coronary sinus and subsequent opacification of the right cardiac chambers. A diagnosis of right coronary artery-coronary sinus fistula was made and corrective operation was accomplished.

An unusual case of coronary artery-coronary sinus fistula was described by Raghib and associates (74). This involved a 23-day-old male infant with aortic atresia, hypoplasia of the left ventricle and premature closure of the foramen ovale (Fig. 40). The only effective channel for escape of blood from the left side of the heart was through a system of myocardial sinusoids that connected with the branches of the left coronary artery, on one hand, and a fistula between the left circumflex artery and the coronary sinus, on the other.

Superior vena cava (Fig. 41a)

A rare form of anomalous communication of a coronary artery is that in which the artery joins the superior vena cava. To our knowledge, only two examples have been reported.

The first case was reported by Gensini and associates (39) in 1966.

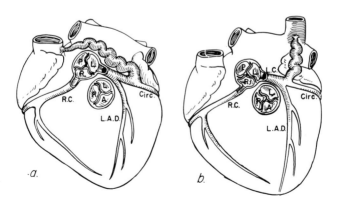

FIG. 41. Anomalous communication of the left circumflex coronary artery with superior venae cavae. a. With right superior vena cava. b. With persistent left superior vena cava.

This was the case of a 53-year-old woman with complaints of palpitations, thoracic pain and dyspnea. A grade III, harsh, to-and-fro, systolic and diastolic murmur was present over the second intercostal space at the right sternal border. Hemodynamic studies revealed a left-to-right shunt to the superior vena cava at about the level of its junction with the right atrium. A selective cineaortogram showed aneurysmal dilatation of the left circumflex coronary artery which communicated with the superior vena cava at about the level of its junction with the right atrium. Findings suggesting the presence of a patent ductus arteriosus accompanied by unusual location of a continuous murmur should raise the suspicion of anomalous communication of a coronary artery.

The second case was reported by Effler and associates (28) in 1967. This concerned a 58-year-old man in whom the left circumflex coronary artery was also involved. Following surgical division of the anomalous communication, angina pectoris, which had been present preoperatively, disappeared.

Persistent left superior vena cava (Fig. 41b)

Somewhat related to the foregoing condition is that in which a coronary artery joins a persistent left superior vena cava. The one reported case of this condition is that of Stansel and Fenn (84).

The report, which appeared in 1964, involved a 35-year-old woman admitted with increasing fatigability and shortness of breath. On auscultation, a grade III/VI continuous murmur was heard in the second and third intercostal spaces along the left sternal border. Cardiac catheterization confirmed the presence of a left-to-right shunt, but the data obtained were nonspecific. A retrograde aortogram demonstrated a large, tortuous left coronary branch communicating with a left persistent superior vena cava. This anomaly was complicated by bacterial infection. After appropriate antibacterial treatment, the patient underwent operation and division of the fistula was carried out successfully.

Pulmonary trunk (Fig. 42)

In the condition under consideration, the two coronary arteries arise normally from the aorta. In addition, one or several arteries that communicate with the normally arising coronary arteries join the pulmonary trunk (6) and provide a route for escape of coronary arterial blood into the pulmonary trunk.

Gobel and associates (41) made an arteriographic study of this con-

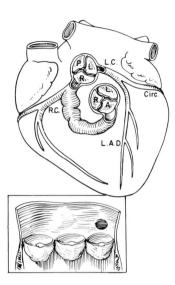

FIG. 42. Anomalous communication of right coronary artery with pulmonary trunk. In this condition, each of the standard coronary arteries arise from the aorta, while the vessel communicating with the pulmonary trunk may be considered an accessory coronary artery. Inset: Ostium of accessory coronary artery in pulmonary trunk.

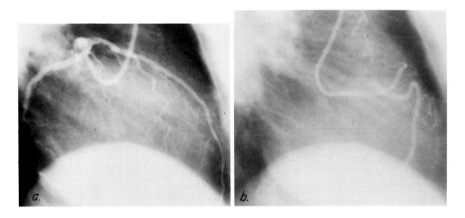

FIG. 43. Anomalous communication of a branch of the right coronary artery with the pulmonary trunk. *a.* Lateral view of selective arteriogram of the left coronary artery. The anterior descending and left circumflex arteries appear normal in this perspective. *b.* Lateral view of selective arteriogram of the right coronary artery. A small branch of the artery communicates with the pulmonary trunk. From ref. 56.

dition. In most of their cases, the anomalous arterial connection with the pulmonary trunk was represented by a plexus of small vessels emptying into the pulmonary artery through several small openings. In one of these cases, two branches (one from the left anterior descending and the other from the right coronary artery) joined in a cavernous mass of vessels lying near the base of the pulmonary artery and emptying into this artery. In another case, a branch of the right coronary artery communicated with an artery arising from the pulmonary trunk (Fig. 43).

In the condition under consideration, the shunt is associated with a continuous murmur. Classically, the murmur is heard at the left sternal border in the same location as the murmur of patent ductus arteriosus. Usually, since the shunts are small, the preferential method for diagnosis

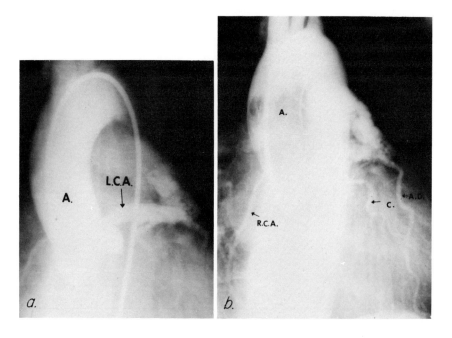

FIG. 44. Aortograms showing anomalous communication of left coronary artery with pulmonary trunk. *a.* Frontal view. In addition to showing the right coronary artery arising from the aorta (A.), this view shows that the left coronary artery (L.C.A.) which is grossly enlarged communicates with the pulmonary trunk as the simultaneous opacification of the left coronary artery and the pulmonary trunk occurs. *b.* Frontal view. From the main left coronary artery, a wide vessel proceeds to the pulmonary trunk, while the circumflex (C.) and anterior descending (A.D.) branches are of normal caliber. From ref. 6.

is selective coronary arteriography. Gobel and associates (41) reported on six cases of shunts between the coronary and pulmonary arteries with normal origin of the coronary arteries. The source for the shunt was the left coronary artery in two of these six cases (Fig. 44), both coronary arteries in three cases and the right coronary artery in one case. The patients may be asymptomatic or may manifest symptoms of myocardial ischemia, heart failure, or both (6, 41, 55, 71).

The justification for surgical interruption of the anomalous connection in this type of case according to Gobel and associates (41) includes relief of symptoms, prophylaxis against complications of coronary artery disease and the prevention of bacterial infection.

Right ventricle (Fig. 45 through 48)

Among the 200 cases of anomalous communications of the coronary arteries reviewed by Oldham and associates (72), there were 78 in which the termination was into the right ventricle. The coronary arterial source was the right coronary artery in 49 cases, the left in 23, both arteries in two cases and branches of a single coronary artery in four cases.

Usually, a continuous murmur is present in these cases unless the right ventricular pressure rises; under this condition, the intensity of the systolic component diminishes. The usual location for the murmur is along the left lower sternal border at the third to fifth intercostal spaces. The part of the right ventricle which most commonly receives the anomalous communication is its outflow tract and, less commonly, its apex. The posterior aspect of the ventricle has also been involved in some cases.

In the case which follows we examined the specimen submitted by Dr. D. D. Tweedale for review (Fig. 45). The patient, a female infant, presented with tachycardia and a murmur was discovered. This child died at the age of 5 weeks and, at necropsy, the anomaly of major interest pertained to the left coronary artery. The great vessels were normally related and the pulmonary trunk appeared slightly larger than the aorta. The left coronary artery was very wide at its origin, measuring about 1 cm in diameter. Shortly after its origin, the artery divided into a lateral and a medial branch. The lateral branch divided in turn into the circumflex and the anterior descending arteries. The medial branch of the main left coronary artery was wide and, after a short course, dipped into the base of the ventricular septum (Fig. 45b). As the artery entered the ventricular septum, it communicated with a chamber-like space lined with endothelium within the anterior part of the ventricular septum. This

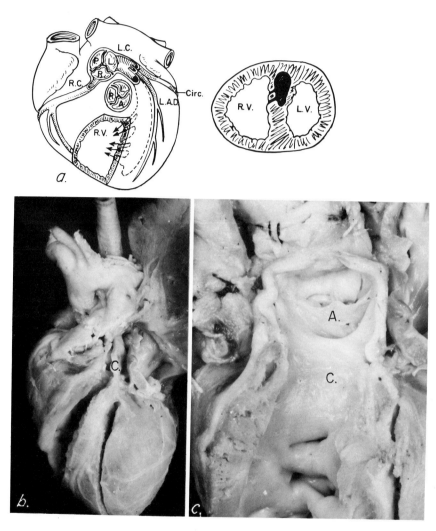

FIG. 45. Multiple anomalous communications of branch of anterior descending coronary artery with right ventricle. *a.* Diagram. *b.* Lateral view of exterior of heart. A wide vessel (C.) arises from the left coronary artery and proceeds to the right of the interventricular sulcus as a wide channel. *c.* Interior of aorta (A.) and the wide channel (C.) leading from the branch of the left coronary artery. Multiple openings in the channel leading to the right ventricle.

space measured 4 by 2 cm and extended from the base of the septum to a point about 2 cm from the apex. Space in the ventricular septum was walled with bundles of cardiac muscle between which there were numerous

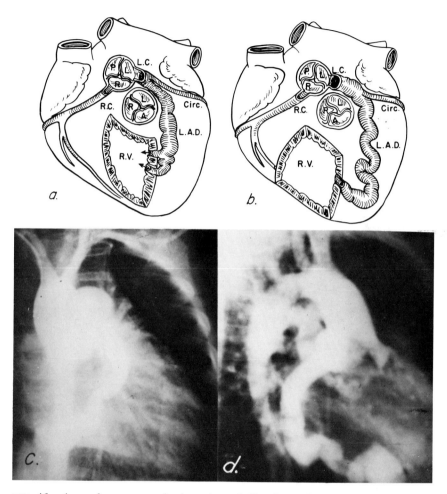

FIG. 46. Anomalous communications (*a* and *b*) of anterior descending coronary artery with right ventricle. *a.* By way of two openings. *b.* By way of one opening. *c* and *d.* Aortograms in a case of anomalous communication of the left coronary artery with the right ventricle. *c.* Frontal view. *d.* Lateral view.

communications with the right ventricle (Fig. 45*c*). The right ventricle was enlarged and hypertrophied; the left ventricular cavity was smaller.

Left atrium (Fig. 49 and 50)

Anomalous communication of a coronary artery with the left side of the heart is very rare. Among the 50 cases of anomalous coronary arterial

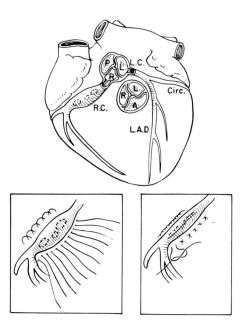

Multiple anomalous communications of right coronary artery with cardiac chamber. Insets: These show the surgical procedure which involves interruption of each of the anomalous branches.

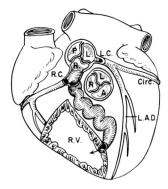

FIG. 48. Anomalous communication of right coronary artery with right ventricle.

communication which we reviewed in 1961, there were three cases in which the anomalous communication was with the left atrium and two in which it was with the left ventricle. In the literature, we found only 24 instances in which a coronary artery communicated with the left side of the heart: the left atrium in 18 cases and the left ventricle in six (2, 8, 9, 14, 17–21, 25, 28, 38, 54, 64, 75, 81).

Mozen (64), in 1956, recognized the first case. In this instance, the left coronary artery was found during operation to join the left atrium for a presumed patent ductus arteriosus. The fistula was successfully closed. Sloman and associates (81), in 1965, reported a case in which the left coronary artery communicated with the pulmonary trunk through its circumflex branch which also communicated with the left atrium.

The clinical history of one of the cases, that of Char and Hara (17), is summarized.

In a five-year-old girl, a continuous murmur was best heard in the first to fourth left intercostal spaces, and the electrocardiographic signs were

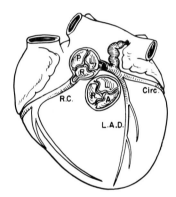

FIG. 49. Anomalous communication of left coronary artery with left atrium.

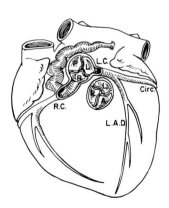

FIG. 50. Anomalous communication of right coronary artery with left atrium.

suggestive of left ventricular preponderance. A thoracic roentgenogram revealed a somewhat enlarged left atrium and left ventricle and apparently normal pulmonary vasculature. Right heart catheterization did not reveal a left-to-right shunt. Retrograde aortography showed a large fistulous tract leading from the aorta to the left atrium. At operation, the left coronary artery was enlarged to a diameter of about 1.2 cm with thinning of its walls. Three and one-half centimeters from its origin, a branch led from the left coronary artery to the left atrium and was aneurysmal. It measured 3 cm in length, 2 cm in width and 1.8 cm in height. The coronary artery distal to the aneurysm was also enlarged. The anomalous branch was obliterated at its origin. The postoperative course of the patient was uneventful.

In the case described by Agusti and associates (8), the patient was a boy, four years and eight months old, in whom a heart murmur had been heard at the age of 18 months. The child was asymptomatic until the age of four years. He then complained of episodic precordial thoracic pain and exhibited mild fatigue on exertion, but had no cyanosis, edema, or other symptoms.

On physical examination, the heart was slightly enlarged and a grade III/VI continuous murmur was heard over the fourth right intercostal space. In addition, an apical holosystolic murmur that was well transmitted to the left axilla was present. The first and second cardiac sounds were normal in intensity and normally split. Cardiac catheterization revealed normal pressures in the right heart chambers and there was no evidence of a left-to-right shunt. Selective aortography revealed that the right coronary artery pursued a tortuous course. Two centimeters from its origin, the artery gave off a branch which passed superiorly and posteriorly to enter the left atrium.

At operation, the proximal portion of the right coronary artery was wide, measuring approximately 6 mm in diameter. The branch, which terminated anomalously, passed near the right atrial appendage and then entered the left atrium. Beyond this branch, the right coronary artery was short. Temporary occlusion of the main right coronary artery did not disturb myocardial function; therefore, it was ligated and divided. The continuous thrill disappeared. Some days after operation, episodes of recurrent anterior thoracic pain unrelated to exercise appeared and lasted 5 to 10 min. The electrocardiogram revealed diaphragmatic myocardial infarction. Laboratory studies, however, were within normal limits.

One year after operation, the patient was admitted to the hospital because of continuing episodes of thoracic pain. Aortography showed a normal left coronary artery. The right coronary artery was only faintly visualized as a large pouch representing that portion of the vessel proximal to the site of surgical interruption. Distal ramifications of the right coronary artery were not visualized. At the age of eight years, the patient manifested thoracic pain of increasing frequency. The electrocardiogram showed decrease in the magnitude of the Q wave in leads III and aVF from that seen in electrocardiograms made shortly after the operation. A multilevel exercise tolerance test was performed with normal results. Selective coronary cineaortography showed no change from the earlier study except for development of collateral vessels.

This case is of specal interest because, as far as we are aware, it is the only reported case in which the right coronary artery joined the left atrium, and also because the patient developed diaphragmatic myocardial infarction after operation.

Left ventricle (Fig. 51 and 52)

Anomalous communication of a coronary artery with the left ventricle is the least common among all forms of coronary arterial cardiac fistula. In the literature we found reports of five cases of anomalous communication of a coronary artery with the left ventricle (29, 37, 57, 60, 89). We encountered an additional example of this condition in a specimen submitted by Dr. Lewis H. Booker for review. Thus six cases were available for analysis. In five of the six cases, the right coronary artery was involved and in the sixth, the anterior descending artery.

A clear description of the clinical features was given in the case reported by Galioto and associates (37), in which the right ventricle com-

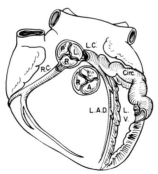

FIG. 51. Anomalous communication of left circumflex coronary artery with left ventricle.

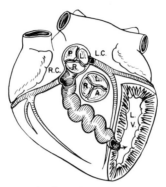

FIG. 52.   Anomalous communication of right coronary artery with left ventricle.

municated with the left ventricle. This concerned a four-year-old boy
with a murmur that was first heard at the age of one year. The child
suffered from frequently occurring upper respiratory infections but had
had no chest pain. On physical examination, a grade III/IV, harsh ejection
systolic murmur was heard over the lower part of the left sternal border;
this was followed by a grade III/VI, decrescendo, diastolic murmur, best
heard at the third left intercostal space and transmitted to the left sternal
border. No thrills were palpable.

An additional case of left anterior descending coronary artery communicating with the left ventricle was reported by Lovitt and Lutz (57).
These authors described a 62-year-old man who died suddenly. At necropsy, the heart was enlarged, weighing 500 g. There was extensive hypertrophy of the left ventricle, which measured 2 cm in thickness. On the
anterior surface of the left ventricle there was a rounded, fibrous protrusion
2 cm in diameter which, on section, revealed a honeycombed cavity filled
with blood. Entering this aneurysm were several branches of the anterior
descending coronary artery. The cavity of the aneurysm communicated
directly with the lumen of the left ventricle.

Another example of congenital fistula of the right coronary artery connected with the left ventricle was described by Eguchi and associates
(29). Their patient, an asymptomatic five-year-old girl, had been found
to have a murmur at the age of two years. Physical examination revealed
a grade III/VI, diastolic, blowing murmur over the entire right side of
the thorax with maximal intensity at the fourth intercostal space to the
right of the sternum.

In two cases, one described by McNamara and Gross (60) and the other by Tanabe and Isomatsu (89), a continuous murmur was noted. In the case described by Eguchi and associates (29) only a diastolic murmur was present. In the case reported by Galioto and co-workers (37) the murmur was described as being systolic and diastolic, but the diastolic murmur was decrescendo. Eguchi and co-workers (29) postulated that the systolic murmur results from systolic ejection of blood from the left ventricle into the coronary artery rather than from blood flowing from the coronary artery into the left ventricle.

The diastolic blood pressure was low in most of the patients described. In McNamara and Gross's case (60) it was 108/58; in Tanabe and Isomatsu's (89), 160/60; in the Eguchi group's case (29), 94/44; and in the Galioto group's (37), 110/60 mm Hg.

Electrocardiographic signs of left ventricular hypertrophy were noted in all cases in which the electrocardiographic findings have been described (29, 37, 60, 89).

All authors emphasize that surgical technique should preserve the continuity of the blood supply in the distal part of the parent coronary artery. In one case of Tanabe and Isomatsu (89), an aneurysmally dilated right coronary artery was closed proximally and distally. No evidence of myocardial ischemia was noted, but the patient died from hemorrhage 15 hours after the operation.

REFERENCES

1. ABBOTT M. Anomalous origin from the pulmonary artery, in: Osler W (Ed), "Osler's modern medicine, its theory and practice." Philadelphia, Lea and Febiger, v 4, 1908, p 420.
2. ABBOTT OA, RIVAROLA CH and LOGUE RB. Surgical correction of coronary arteriovenous fistula. *J Thorac Cardiovasc Surg* **42**: 660, 1961.
3. ABRAMS LD, EVANS DW and HOWARTH FH. Coronary artery-right ventricular fistula treated surgically. *Br Heart J* **29**: 132, 1967.
4. ALEXANDER WS and GREEN HC. Coronary blood vessel arising from cardiac ventricle: Report of a case showing other cardiac anomalies. *Arch Pathol* **53**: 187, 1952.
5. ALLANBY KD, BRINTON WD, CAMPBELL M and GARDNER F. Pulmonary atresia and the collateral circulation to the lungs. *Guys Hosp Rep* **99**: 110, 1950.
6. AMPLATZ K, AGUIRRE J and LILLEHEI CW. Coronary arteriovenous fistula into main pulmonary artery. *JAMA* **172**: 1384, 1960.
7. ARAYA I, ODO Y, YAMANOTO K et al. Surgical experience with congenital coronary arteriovenous fistula. *Jap J Thorac Surg* **19**: 281, 1966.
8. AGUSTI R, LIEBMAN J, ANKENEY J, MACLEOD CA, LINTON DS and WILTSIE R. Congenital right coronary artery to left atrium fistula. *Am J Cardiol* **19**: 428, 1967.
9. BAYLIS JH and CAMPBELL M. An unusual cause for a continuous murmur *Guys Hosp Rep* **101**: 174, 1952.
10. BERMAN DA, ALEXANDER CS, ADICOFF A and SAKO Y. Coronary arterio-

venous fistula: Report of an unusual case simulating atrial septal defect. *Am J Cardiol* **15**: 853, 1964.

11. BJÖRCK G and CRAFOORD C. Arteriovenous aneurysm on the pulmonary artery simulating patent ductus arteriosus Botalli. *Thorax* **2**: 65, 1947.
12. BJÖRK VO and BJÖRK L. Coronary artery fistula. *J Thorac Cardiovasc Surg* **49**: 921, 1965.
13. BLAKEWAY H. A hitherto undescribed malformation of the heart. *J Anat Physiol* **52**: 354, 1918.
14. BOSHER LH JR, VASLI S, McCUE CM and BELTER LF. Congenital coronary arteriovenous fistula associated with large patent ductus. *Circulation* **20**: 254, 1959.
15. BROOKS H ST J. Two cases of an abnormal coronary artery of the heart arising from the pulmonary artery: With some remarks upon the effect of this anomaly in producing cirsoid dilatation of the vessels. *J Anat Physiol* **20**: 26, 1886.
16. BROWN RC and BURNETT JD. Anomalous channel between aorta and right ventricle: Report of a case. *Pediatrics* **3**: 597, 1949.
17. CHAR F and HARA M. Congenital coronary artery fistula. Communication of the left coronary artery with the left atrium. *J Lancet* **86**: 93, 1966.
18. COLBECK JC and SHAW JM. Coronary aneurysm with arteriovenous fistula. *Am Heart J* **48**: 270, 1954.
19. COOLEY DA and ELLIS PR JR. Surgical considerations of coronary arterial fistula. *Am J Cardiol* **10**: 467, 1962.
20. COOLEY DA. Discussion of Effler DB et al. (28).
21. CROOM RD III, WILCOX BR and ABNEY RL III. Right coronary artery—coronary sinus arteriovenous fistula. *Ann Thorac Surg* **4**: 182, 1967.
22. DAVIS C JR, DILLON RF, FELL EH and GASUL BM. Anomalous coronary artery simulating patent ductus arteriosus. *JAMA* **160**: 1047, 1956.
23. DAVISON PH, McCRACKEN BH and McILVEEN DJS. Congenital coronary arterio-venous aneurysm. *Br Heart J* **17**: 569, 1955.
24. DEDICHEN H, SKALLEBERG L and CHAPPELEN C JR. Congenital coronary artery fistula. *Thorax* **21**: 121, 1966.
25. DIEHL A. Quoted by Gasul BM et al. (38).
26. EDWARDS JE, GLADDING TC and WEIR AB JR. Congenital communication between the right coronary artery and right atrium. *J Thorac Surg* **35**: 662, 1968.
27. EDWARDS JE. Anomalous coronary arteries with special reference to arterio-venous-like communications. *Circulation* **17**: 1001, 1958.
28. EFFLER DB, SHELDON WC, TURNER JJ and GROVES LK. Coronary arterio-venous fistulas: Diagnosis and surgical management. Report of fifteen cases. *Surgery* **61**: 41, 1967.
29. EGUCHI S, NITTA H, ASSANO K, TANAKA M and HOSHINO K. Congenital fistula of the right coronary artery to the left ventricle. The third case in the literature. *Am Heart J* **80**: 242, 1970.
30. EMMINGER E. Arterio-venöses Aneurysma der rechten Herzkranschlagader. *Klin Med* 2: 652, 1947.
31. ENGLE MA, GOLDSMITH EI, HOLSWADE GR, GOLDBERG HP and GLENN F. Congenital coronary arteriovenous fistula. Diagnostic evaluation and surgical correction. *N Engl J Med* **264**: 856, 1961.
32. ESPINO VELA J, VALAZQUEZ T and FUENMAYOR A. Ampila comunicación congenita de la aorta con el ventriculo derecho a traves de la arteria coronaria derecha anomala. *Arch Inst Cardiol Mex* **21**: 686, 1951.
33. ESSENBERG JM. An anomalous left coronary artery in human fetus: Its passage through the left atrium and possible discharge into the right atrium. *Anat Rec* **108**: 709, 1950.
34. FELL EH, WEINBERG M JR, GORDON AS, GASUL BM and JOHNSON FR. Surgery for congenital coronary artery arteriovenous fistulae. *Arch Surg* **77**: 331, 1958.

35. FORSTMANN W and GEISSLER W. Über die arteriovenösen Fisteln der Koronararterien. *Fortschr Geb Roentgenstr Nuklearmed* **93**: 143, 1960.
36. FRASER RS, LOGAN L and BALFOUR GS. Aneurysm of the right coronary artery. Rupture into the right atrium with survival for one year. *Am J Cardiol* **6**: 830, 1960.
37. GALIOTO FM JR, REITMAN MJ, SLOVIS AJ and SAROT IA. Right coronary artery to left ventricle fistula. A case report and discussion. *Am Heart J* **82**: 93, 1971.
38. GASUL BM, ARCILLA RA, FELL EH, LYNFIELD J, BICOFF JP and LUAN LL. Congenital coronary arteriovenous fistula. Clinical, phonocardiographic, angiocardiographic and hemodynamic studies in five patients. *Pediatrics* **25**: 531, 1960.
39. GENSINI GG, PALACIO A and BUONANNO C. Fistula from circumflex coronary artery to superior vena cava. *Circulation* **33**: 297, 1966.
40. GERISCH RA, DODRILL FD, CAROMONEY WJ and KRABBENHOFT KL. Anomalous coronary artery communicating with right atrium; case report. *Harper Hosp Bull* **21**: 515, 1963.
41. GOBEL FL, ANDERSON CF, BALTAXE HA, AMPLATZ K and WANG Y. Shunts between the coronary and pulmonary arteries with normal origin of the coronary arteries. *Am J Cardiol* **25**: 655, 1970.
42. GRANT RT. Development of the cardiac coronary vessels in the rabbit. *Heart* **13**: 261, 1926.
43. GRANT RP, SANDERS RJ, MORROW AG and BRAUNWALD E. Symposium on diagnostic methods in the study of left-to-right shunts. *Circulation* **16**: 791, 1957.
44. HABERMAN JH, HOWARD ML and JOHNSON ES. Rupture of the coronary sinus with hemopericardium: A rare complication of coronary arteriovenous fistula. *Circulation* **28**: 1143, 1963.
45. HALLER JA JR and LITTLE JA. Diagnosis and surgical correction of congenital coronary artery-coronary sinus fistula. *Circulation* **27**: 939, 1963.
46. HALLMAN GL, COOLEY DA and SINGER DB. Congenital anomalies of the coronary arteries: Anatomy, pathology and surgical treatment. *Surgery* **59**: 133, 1966.
47. HALPERT B. Arteriovenous communication between the right coronary artery and the coronary sinus. *Heart* **15**: 129, 1930.
48. HARRIS PN. Aneurysmal dilatation of the cardiac coronary arteries: Review of the literature and report of a case. *Am J Pathol* **13**: 89, 1937.
49. HONEY M. Coronary arterial fistula. *Br Heart J* **26**: 719, 1964.
50. HUDSPETH AS. Discussion. *J Thorac Cardiovasc Surg* **53**: 92, 1967.
51. JOHNSON J. Quoted by Davis C Jr et al. (22).
52. KIMBIRIS D, KASPARIAN H, KNIBBE P and BREST AN. Coronary artery-coronary sinus fistula. *Am J Cardiol* **26**: 532, 1970.
53. KITIYAKARA K, JUMBALA B and SUKROJANA K. Congenital fistula between a coronary artery and the right atrium: Report of a case successfully treated by open heart surgery. *Acta Chir Scand* **129**: 663, 1965.
54. KITTLE CF. Discussion. *Arch Surg* **78**: 204, 1959.
55. KNOBLICH R and RAWSON AJ. Arteriovenous fistula of the heart. *Am Heart J* **52**: 474, 1956.
56. LEE GB, GOBEL FL, LILLEHEI CW, NEFF WS and ELIOT RS. Correction of shunt from right conal coronary artery to pulmonary trunk with relief of symptoms. *Circulation* **37**: 244, 1968.
57. LOVITT WV JR and LUTZ S JR. Embryological aneurysm of the myocardial vessels. *Arch Pathol* **57**: 163, 1954.
58. LÖWENHEIM K. Eine seltene Missbildung der Coronargefässe. *Frankfurt Z Path* **43**: 63, 1932.
59. MCINTOSH HD, SLEEPER JC, THOMPSON HK JR, SEALY WC and YOUNG WG JR. Preoperative evaluation of a continuous murmur in the chest. *Arch Surg* **82**: 74, 1961.

60. McNamara JJ and Gross RE. Congenital coronary artery fistula. *Surgery* **65**: 59, 1969.
61. Michaud P, Froment R, Viard H, Gravier J and Verney RN. Les fistules coronaire-ventriculaires droites. *Arch Mal Coeur* **56**: 143, 1963.
62. Michel D and Herbst M. Über eine ungewöhnliche Anomalie der Koronararterie. *Z Kreislaufforsch* **46**: 538, 1957.
63. Morrow AG. Quoted by Edwards JE et al. (26).
64. Mozen HE. Congenital cirsoid aneurysm of a coronary artery with associated arterio-atrial fistula, treated by operation. A case report. *Ann Surg* **144**: 215, 1956.
65. Muir CS. Coronary arterio-cameral fistula. *Br Heart J* **22**: 374, 1960.
66. Munkner T, Petersen O and Vesterdal J. Congenital aneurysm of the coronary artery with an arteriovenous fistula. *Acta Radiol (Stockh)* **50**: 333, 1958.
67. Murray RH. Single coronary artery with fistulous communication: Report of 2 cases. *Circulation* **28**: 437, 1963.
68. Nagayo M and Takahashi. Aneurysma serpentinum der linken Koronararterie. *J Jap Assoc Pathol* **22**: 583, 1932.
69. Neill C and Mounsey P. Auscultation in patent ductus arteriosus: With a description of two fistulae simulating patent ductus. *Br Heart J* **20**: 61, 1958.
70. Neufeld HN, Lester RG, Adams P Jr, Anderson RC, Lillehei CW and Edwards JE. Congenital communication of a coronary artery with a cardiac chamber or the pulmonary trunk ("coronary artery fistula"). *Circulation* **24**: 171, 1961.
71. Noonan JA and Spencer FC. Single coronary artery with coronary arteriovenous fistula communicating with the right ventricle. *Am J Cardiol* **15**: 848, 1965.
72. Oldham HN Jr, Ebert PA, Young WG and Sabiston DC Jr. Surgical management of congenital coronary artery fistula. *Ann Thorac Surg* **12**: 503, 1971.
73. Paul O, Sweet RH and White PD. Coronary arteriovenous fistula: Case report. *Am Heart J* **37**: 441, 1949.
74. Raghib G, Bloemendaal RD, Kanjuh VI and Edwards JE. Aortic atresia and premature closure of foramen ovale. Myocardial sinusoids and coronary arteriovenous fistula serving as outflow channel. *Am Heart J* **70**: 476, 1965.
75. Reed WA and Kittle CF. Congenital coronary artery fistula. *Arch Surg* **93**: 772, 1966.
76. Sabiston DC Jr, Ross RS, Criley JM, Gaertner RA, Neill CA and Taussig HB. Surgical management of congenital lesions of the coronary circulation. *Ann Surg* **157**: 908, 1963.
77. Sakakibara S, Yokoyama M, Takao A, Nogi M and Gomi H. Coronary arteriovenous fistula. Nine operated cases. *Am Heart J* **72**: 307, 1966.
78. Sanger PW, Taylor FH and Robicsek F. The diagnosis and treatment of coronary arteriovenous fistula. *Surgery* **45**: 344, 1959.
79. Schaffer AB, St Ville J and Mackler SA. Coronary arteriovenous fistula with patent ductus. *Am Heart J* **65**: 758, 1963.
80. Scott DH. Aneurysm of the coronary arteries. *Am Heart J* **36**: 403, 1948.
81. Sloman G, Macphee A and Fairley K. An unusual coronary arterio-cameral fistula. *Am J Cardiol* **15**: 856, 1965.
82. Sondergaard T. Henry Ford Hosp Intern Symp Cardiovasc Surgery. Philadelphia, WB Saunders, 1955, 490 pp.
83. Sones FM and Shirey EK. Cine coronary arteriography. *Mod Concepts Cardiovasc Dis* **31**: 735, 1962.
84. Stansel HC Jr and Fenn JE. Coronary arteriovenous fistula between the left coronary artery and persistent left superior vena cava complicated by bacterial endocarditis. *Ann Surg* **160**: 292, 1964.
85. Stephenson HE. Discussion of Effler DB et al. (28).
86. Swan H, Wilson JN, Woodwark G and Blount SG Jr. Surgical oblitera-

tion of a coronary artery fistula to right ventricle. *Arch Surg* **79**: 820, 1959.

87. SYMBAS PN, SCHLANT RC, HATCHER CR JR and LINDSAY J.   Congenital fistula of right coronary artery to right ventricle complicated by Actinobacillus actinomycetemcomitans endarteritis. *J Thorac Cardiovasc Surg* **53**: 379, 1967.

88. TABER RE, GALE HH and LAM CR. Coronary artery-right heart fistulas. *J Thorac Cardiovasc Surg* **53**: 84, 1967.

89. TANABE T and ISOMATSU T.   Tortuous right coronary fistula to the left ventricle. *J Jap Assoc Thorac Surg* **10**: 519, 1962.

90. TREVOR RS.   Aneurysm of the descending branch of the right coronary artery. *Proc R Soc Med* **5**: 20, 1912.

91. TSAGARIS TJ and HECHT HH.   Coronary artery aneurysm and subacute bacterial endarteritis. *Ann Intern Med* **57**: 116, 1962.

92. UPSHAW CB JR.   Congenital coronary arteriovenous fistula. Report of a case with an analysis of seventy-three reported cases. *Am Heart J* **63**: 399, 1962. *Proc R Soc Med* **5**: 20, 1912.

93. VALDIVIA E, ROWE GG and ANGEVINE DM.   Large congenital aneurysm of the right coronary artery. *Arch Pathol* **63**: 163, 1957.

94. WALTHER RJ, STARKEY GWB, ZERVOPOLUS E and GIBBONS GA. Coronary arteriovenous fistula: Clinical and physiologic report on two patients, with review of the literature. *Am J Med* **22**: 213, 1957.

95. WATSON H.   "Pediatric cardiology." St. Louis, CB Mosby Co, 1968.

96. WEDELL HG and TELOH HA.   Congenital communication between the right coronary artery and right atrium. *Quart Bull Northw Univ Med Sch* **33**: 285, 1959.

97. YENEL F.   Coronary arteriovenous communication. Report of a case and review of the literature. *N Engl J Med* **265**: 577, 1961.

CHAPTER VIII

ANOMALOUS ORIGIN OF THE CORONARY ARTERIES FROM THE PULMONARY TRUNK

INCIDENCE

Anomalous origin of the left coronary artery from the pulmonary artery was initially described by Abbott (1) in 1908. Her case involved a 64-year-old woman. Abrikossoff (2) reported a case in 1911, that of a five-month-old female infant. In 1933, Bland and associates (12) described the clinical picture in this anomaly. The ratio of females to males was considered to be 2:1 by George and Knowlan (35). This is a rare congenital anomaly and the incidence of this lesion among all types of congenital heart disease is somewhere between 0.25% and 0.50%, that is, between 1 in 200 and 1 in 400.

EMBRYOLOGY

The coronary arteries arise as solid angioblastic buds which are visible before truncoconal partitioning is complete. These then extend rapidly

[78]

through the epicardium. The left coronary artery makes a sharp turn from its origin as it descends into the conoventricular groove. Division into the anterior descending and circumflex branches occurs within the groove by the middle of the seventh week of gestation. The right coronary artery emerges into the depression between the right atrium and the conus giving off branches as it extends along the atrioventricular sulcus to the dorsal aspect of the heart. The smaller branches of the coronary arteries develop into a rich capillary network and connect through a plexus with the coronary sinus. Some small branches of the coronary arteries communicate with muscular intertrabecular spaces which are relatively large early in cardiac development, especially in the right ventricular wall. The high incidence of coronary abnormalities accompanying gross truncoconal malformations is understandable since the development of the coronary arteries occurs practically simultaneously with partitioning of the truncus and the conus.

From an anatomic point of view, five types of anomalous origins of the coronary arteries from the pulmonary arteries occur: 1) origin of the left coronary artery itself or a branch of it from the pulmonary artery, 2) origin of the right coronary artery from the pulmonary artery, 3) origin of both coronary arteries from the pulmonary artery, 4) origin of a single coronary artery from the pulmonary artery and 5) origin of accessory coronary artery(ies) from the pulmonary artery (same as communication of a coronary artery with pulmonary trunk; see Chapter VII).

ANOMALOUS ORIGIN OF THE LEFT CORONARY ARTERY FROM THE PULMONARY ARTERY (FIG. 53 AND 54)

Pathologic Anatomy

In this anomaly, the left coronary artery arises from the pulmonary arterial system, usually from the pulmonary trunk but rarely from its primary branches (23, 48, 55, 69, 77, 89). The right coronary artery arises in normal fashion from the right aortic sinus and follows a normal course and distibution. In most cases of this anomaly, the main left coronary artery originates from the left pulmonary sinus (Fig. 53) and is usually much shorter than normal, measuring 2 to 5 mm in length before bifurcation. This may pose some technical problems at operation when ligation is undertaken. In some instances the right coronary artery is dilated and tortuous (14) (Fig. 55). Grossly visible anastomotic vessels between the right and left coronary arteries were described by Case and associates (18)

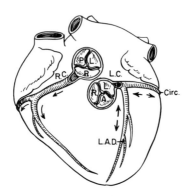

FIG. 53. Anomalous origin of the left coronary artery from the pulmonary trunk. A stage in early infancy is shown when there may be little or no flow through the anomalous vessel. Perfusion from the pulmonary artery may be present at this stage.

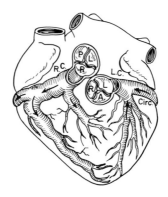

FIG. 54. Anomalous origin of the left coronary artery from the pulmonary trunk. In the stage shown, extensive collaterals have developed between the two coronary arteries allowing blood derived from the right coronary artery ultimately to enter the pulmonary trunk by way of the anomalously arising left coronary artery.

and by Moller and associates (68) (Fig. 54). Anastomotic communications have also been demonstrated by several authors by postmortem injections (6, 18, 20, 53, 84, 86, 97, 104). The left ventricle is usually markedly dilated and hypertrophied (Fig. 56). Endocardial fibroelastosis of variable degree is present in the left ventricle in all cases (Fig. 57a and b). In some instances, both ventricles show endocardial fibroelastosis. Usman

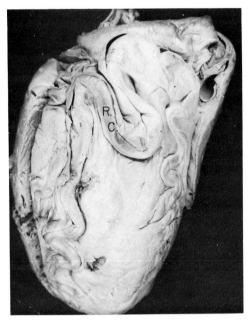

FIG. 55. Right lateral view of heart in a case of anomalous origin of the left coronary artery from the pulmonary trunk. The right coronary artery (R.C.) is grossly enlarged and tortuous. The left coronary artery is similarly enlarged.

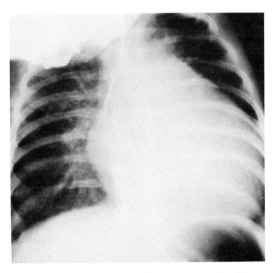

FIG. 56. Roentgenogram of thorax of a 10-week-old girl with anomalous origin of the left coronary artery from the pulmonary trunk. The heart is enlarged.

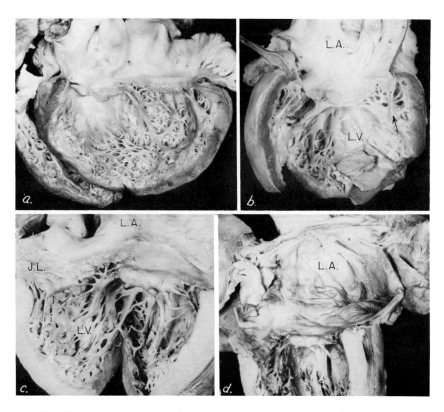

FIG. 57. Pathologic features in three cases of anomalous origin of the left coronary artery from the pulmonary trunk. *a.* Major dilatation of the left ventricle associated with endocardial fibroelastosis and subendocardial scarring of left ventricular myocardium. From a 10-week-old girl. *b.* Left atrium (L.A.) and left ventricle (L.V.). The posteromedial papillary muscle (arrow) of the left ventricle shows atrophy on the basis of infarction. The related free wall of the left ventricle shows subendocardial scarring. Fibroelastosis is also present. From a seven-month-old boy. *c* and *d.* From a seven-year-old girl. *c.* The papillary muscles of the left ventricle (L.V.) show major atrophy on the basis of infarction. Jet lesions (J.L.) are present on the wall of the left atrium (L.A.). *d.* Major dilatation of the left atrium (L.A.) secondary to mitral insufficiency.

and associates (107) described additional calcification of the mitral valve combined with mitral regurgitation in an adult patient. George and Knowlan (35) have reported associated fusion of mitral valve leaflets and shortening of the chordae tendineae in an adult patient.

In the distribution of the left coronary artery, the endocardial aspect of the left ventricular wall often shows recent infarcts and areas of diffuse myocardial fibrosis (56, 61). Calcification may be present in fibrotic areas. Involvement of the papillary muscles has been described and, in some instances, both papillary muscles are involved (Fig. 57b and d) (53, 75, 114). Extensive ventricular scarring may, at times, result in aneurysmal dilatation of the left ventricle (Fig. 57a). Mural thrombi attached to the endocardium of the left ventricle have been described in several cases (17, 41, 43, 99). Vettermarks (109), in 1965, described a recent embolus to the right coronary artery.

The left atrium may be enlarged in association with thickening of its wall (Fig. 57c). A jet lesion involving the left atrial wall, as an expression of mitral regurgitation, may be identified in some instances (Fig. 57d). In three of the cases described by Noren and associates (75) the papillary muscles appeared to take their origin higher from the left ventricular wall than normal and the chordae were correspondingly short.

The most consistent changes are found in the left ventricular papillary muscles, particularly the posteromedial one (Fig. 58a and b), in which acute infarction or scarring and foci of calcific deposits may be identified.

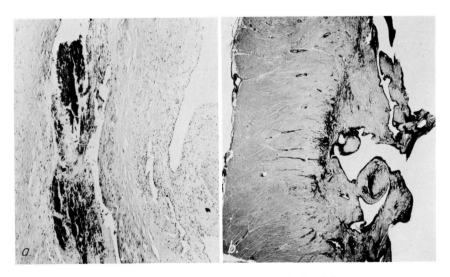

FIG. 58. Photomicrographs of anomalous origin of the left coronary artery from the pulmonary trunk. a. Infarction of posteromedial papillary muscle. Gross specimen in this case is shown in Figure 57b. Hematoxylin and eosin; × 11.5. b. The dark zones represent scarring from subendocardial myocardial infarction. Elastic tissue stain; × 3.5. Gross specimen in this case is shown in Figure 57c and d.

In some cases the anterior papillary muscle may also be scarred (30, 31, 45, 51, 53, 75, 115). These findings are similar to those described by Phillips and associates (79).

The changes of the papillary muscles were found in one adult patient in whom the anterior papillary muscle and its chordae tendineae were completely calcified and looked like a bizarre rock formation (25).

Burchell and Brown (15), in 1962, and Talner and associates (104), in 1965, described cases associated with mitral insufficiency in which extensive myocardial fibrosis and dilatation of the left ventricle and the mitral orifice were present (67). Left ventricular involvement, however, is limited to the apical area in most instances.

Several cases have been reported in which an infant or a child died suddenly (29). In some of these, death was associated with exercise. Postmortem examination after sudden death in these cases showed large, tortuous right coronary arteries (38, 44, 54, 63, 91, 92, 115). The right coronary artery in such cases supplied the posterior wall of both ventricles, and in the cases reported by Ruddock and Stehly (92), Helpern (44) and Gouley (38) the lateral wall of the left ventricle as well. Fibrosis of the myocardium at the subendocardial area frequently involved one-third to one-half of the myocardium in these cases.

Anomalous origin of the left coronary artery from the pulmonary artery is usually not associated with other malformations. In a few cases, however, other cardiovascular malformations have been reported. A patent ductus arteriosus has been reported in a few instances (5, 50, 98). Sabiston and associates (98) described a case associated with ventricular septal defect and Hallman and associates (40) described one case of persistent truncus arteriosus in which the left coronary artery arose from the left pulmonary artery. Masel (64) reported on a patient with tetralogy of Fallot in whom the left coronary artery arose from the right pulmonary artery. Gonzalez-Angulo (37) and Losekoot and their associates (62) described cases in which ventricular septal defect was an associated lesion.

In a patient described by Rao and co-workers (83), the left coronary artery arose from the right pulmonary artery (Fig. 59a and b). The patient was a three-year-old girl with a ventricular septal defect and pulmonary hypertension. On physical examination, the child presented clinical signs of poor development with tachypnea, tachycardia and hepatomegaly. Physical examination revealed a grade III/VI diastolic murmur along the left sternal border. The second sound of the pulmonary area was ac-

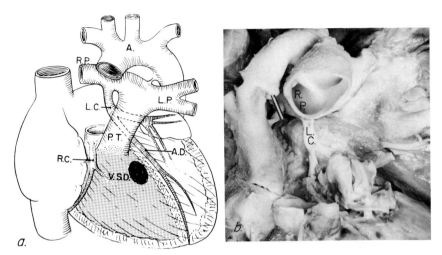

FIG. 59. Anomalous origin of the left coronary artery from the right pulmonary artery in a three-year-old girl with ventricular septal defect (V.S.D.). *a.* Diagram of the basic conditions. *b.* The left coronary artery (L.C.) arises from the right pulmonary artery (R.P.). Probe in aortic end of divided patent ductus arteriosus. From ref. 83.

centuated. Roentgenography of the thorax revealed increased pulmonary vasculature and cardiomegaly. The clinical diagnosis of ventricular septal defect was confirmed by cardiac catheterization, showing left-to-right shunt of 58% at the ventricular level. Cineaortography and selective right ventriculography failed to reveal any abnormal vascular connection. Surgical closure of the ventricular septal defect was followed by death immediately after the operation.

At necropsy, a large ventricular septal defect was found that had been closed with a Teflon patch. The right coronary artery arose normally from the right aortic sinus and followed a normal course and distribution. The left coronary artery arose from the inferior aspect of the right pulmonary artery at a point about 1 cm distal to the bifurcation of the pulmonary trunk. The orifice of the vessel was about 1 mm in diameter. The anomalous vessel coursed inferiorly between the pulmonary arterial trunk and left atrium for a distance of about 1.5 cm and then bifurcated into the anterior descending and circumflex branches. There was no evidence of recent or old myocardial infarction, and histologic examination revealed only a minimal subendocardial scarring of the left ventricle.

In a situation where a large ventricular septal defect is present, the

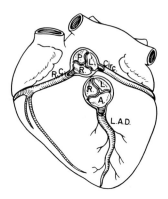

FIG. 60.   Origin of anterior descending coronary artery from the pulmonary trunk. The left circumflex artery arises from the left aortic sinus.

elevated pulmonary arterial pressure helps to propel blood into the anomalous coronary artery, thereby supplying nearly normal perfusion pressure in the myocardial vascular bed (42). Stimulus for the development of collaterals within the two coronary arteries is either absent or of minor proportion, since the pressure in the pulmonary arteries is near systemic levels. If pulmonary arterial pressure falls upon closure of the ventricular septal defect in such cases, a deficiency in perfusion of the myocardium appears. The authors who described this case postulated that after surgical closure of the ventricular septal defect, myocardial ischemia occurred. Similar complications appeared in a case described by Feldt and associates (32) in which a single coronary artery arose from the pulmonary artery.

A variation of anomalous origin of the left coronary artery from the pulmonary artery has been described in three patients. In the cases of Liebman and associates (58) and in that of Schwartz and Robicsek (102), the right coronary artery originated from the right aortic sinus and had a normal root course and distribution. From the left aortic sinus, a small artery arose. This vessel pursued the courses typical for the left circumflex coronary artery. The anterior descending coronary arose from the pulmonary trunk (Fig. 60).

Another variation was described by Edwards (26). There the anterior descending artery arose from the pulmonary trunk, while independent origins of the left circumflex and right coronary arteries were situated in the right aortic sinus.

Clinical Features

The course and diagnosis of anomalous origin of the left coronary system depend on the adequacy of the collateral circulation between the two coronary arteries (Fig. 61). In fetal life, large intercoronary channels are present in the heart and the persistence of these channels after birth may permit adequate perfusion of the left ventricular myocardium. During fetal life, pressures in the pulmonary artery and the aorta are similar and the left ventricular myocardium can be adequately perfused from the pulmonary artery. With the drop of the pulmonary arterial pressure after birth, however, inadequate perfusion through the anomalous left coronary artery may occur. In instances in which the intercoronary anastomoses that are well developed naturally during fetal life become enlarged after birth, the left coronary artery may be perfused from the right coronary artery. The direction of flow, as has been pointed out by Edwards (26), is from the aorta through the coronary system into the pulmonary artery.

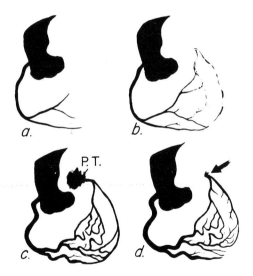

FIG. 61. Functional states in origin of left coronary artery from the pulmonary trunk. *a.* The aorta and its right coronary arterial branch are shown. *b.* Collaterals are developing between the right coronary and left coronary systems. *c.* Collaterals between the right and left coronary systems have developed to the point wherein the pulmonary trunk (P.T.) receives blood from the coronary arterial system. *d.* Following ligation of the anomalously arising left coronary artery, all of the right coronary blood is distributed to the myocardium, since the arteriovenous fistula has been obliterated.

Gasul and associates (34) considered the mortality in this anomaly to be very high (about 80 to 85%). Wesselhoeft and co-workers (112) found that of 140 cases collected from the literature, 116 or 82% were diagnosed in infancy and 24 or 18% in childhood or at an older age.

Symptoms

Symptoms usually begin in infancy. These include discomfort during or after feeding accompanied by dyspnea, tachypnea, pallor, paroxysmal crying and restlessness. Between the angina-like episodes the infant is usually free of symptoms, although dyspnea of varying degree or tachypnea may be observed (111).

The picture then becomes progressive. The episodes increase in frequency and severity. There are frequent upper respiratory infections. Cyanosis, however, is infrequent and, when present, is transient. Rate of growth is slowed in some patients. Signs of congestive heart failure also appear early in infancy. In those patients who survive into childhood these symptoms may diminish in intensity. Sudden death has been observed in some patients during periods of irritability and dyspnea, and in others during induction of anesthesia in preparation for operation or at the time of cardiac catheterization.

One patient, a three-year-old child described by Nora and associates (74), was considered to have been entirely asymptomatic although a murmur of mitral insufficiency, cardiomegaly, and electrocardiographic evidence of myocardial infarction were discovered on a routine physical examination.

Physical Examination

The physical examinations frequently show prominence of the left side of the precordium. Cardiomegaly is present in all patients. The heart sounds are usually normal, but a prominent third sound may occasionally be heard.

Commonly, an ejection type of systolic murmur of grade I to II intensity is present, even in infancy. The murmur seems to be more prominent in patients with associated mitral insufficiency. In the latter circumstance, the murmur is apical and pansystolic and has the qualities of transmission characteristic of that in mitral insufficiency. Uncommonly, a continuous murmur or associated systolic and diastolic murmurs may be heard.

Wesselhoeft and associates (112), reviewing the literature, found murmurs of the type mentioned in nine patients (4, 13, 50, 58, 59, 64), including children and adults (ages ranged from three to 29 years). Most patients appeared to be in good health, and all had normal peripheral pulses and pulse pressures (4, 58). Two of the patients who were poorly developed reported episodes of angina. In each, this symptom disappeared with ligation of the anomalous left coronary artery.

In four other cases that have been reported (10, 31, 50, 57, 81), continuous murmurs simulated the murmur of patent ductus arteriosus in that the continuous murmur was located along the left sternal border. When the murmurs were described as systolic and diastolic, the location was either in the pulmonary area (59, 65) or along the left sternal border (4, 58). Agustsson and associates (3, 4) postulated that the continuous murmur originated within the dilated right coronary artery because of the markedly increased blood flow. It is also likely that the continuous murmur may originate at the site of origin of the left coronary artery. As in patients with coronary arteriovenous fistulae, intracardiac phonocardiography demonstrated that the murmur was present at the termination of the fistula (66). Support for this location also comes from observations at operation when the maximal thrill could be felt at the fistulous termination. Use of intracardiac phonocardiography has not been reported in cases of anomalous left coronary artery, to our knowledge. At operations, however, a thrill has been detected over the pulmonary artery near the entrance of the left coronary artery.

Electrocardiogram

The electrocardiographic characteristics of anomalous left coronary artery were first described by Bland and associates (12). They emphasized that the electrocardiogram was the most useful tool available to make the diagnosis. It is of special importance in the differential diagnosis of cardiomegaly and congestive heart failure in infancy.

In anomalous left coronary artery, a pattern of anterolateral infarction characterized by deep Q waves followed by tall R waves and inverted or diphasic T waves in leads I, aVL, V_5 and V_6 is common (Fig. 62). Occasionally, an elevated ST segment in the left precordial leads may be observed over an extended period, suggesting left ventricular aneurysm. Electrocardiographic evidence of left ventricular hypertrophy, based on prominent posteriorly directed forces, is also a part of the classical electrocardiographic picture of this malformation. In two patients, aged six and seven years, Noren and associates (75) observed a change in the electro-

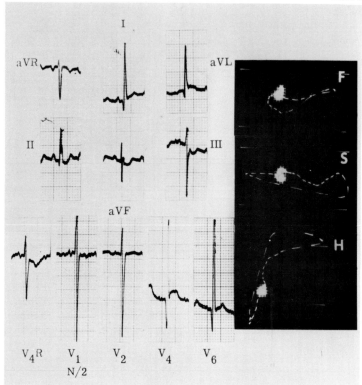

FIG. 62. Characteristic electrocardiographic and vectorcardiographic findings in anomalous origin of the left coronary artery from the pulmonary trunk. The electrocardiogram shows a picture consistent with anterolateral myocardial infarction. In the horizontal plane of the vectorcardiogram, features of anterolateral myocardial infarction are also apparent. Same case as illustrated in Figure 57a.

cardiographic picture which was characterized by the absence of Q waves in lead I, presence of Q waves in lead aVL and abnormal T waves in leads aVL and V_6. With time, classical changes of myocardial infarction may yield to less specific patterns.

Vectorcardiogram

Vectorcardiograms (Fig. 62) show the typical pattern characteristic of anterolateral myocardial infarction and left ventricular hypertrophy. The horizontal plane is especially useful in the diagnosis of anomalous origin of the left coronary artery from the pulmonary artery since it shows that the major portion of the loop is oriented posteriorly and to the left and its direction is clockwise in contrast to the normal direction which is counterclockwise. The picture is similar to the one seen in adult patients with anterolateral myocardial infarction (76).

Roentgenographic Findings

In infants, the roentgenographic features are those of marked cardiomegaly with prominent pulmonary vasculature (36). Mild left atrial enlargement may be present. In some instances signs of pulmonary venous hypertension, such as Kerley lines, may be observed. In older children the cardiomegaly is less striking and left atrial enlargement is usually absent. This is especially so in patients without significant mitral insufficiency. Reduction of cardiac size as a gradually evolving process has been observed in those patients who have been followed for several years.

Angiocardiography and aortography may be of considerable diagnostic help (Fig. 63a). Selective aortography shows evidence of a single coronary artery arising from the aorta in the usual position of the right coronary artery. The vessel may be enlarged and tortuous. In some examinations, retrograde opacification of the left coronary artery after filling of the right coronary artery may be visualized, followed by opacification of

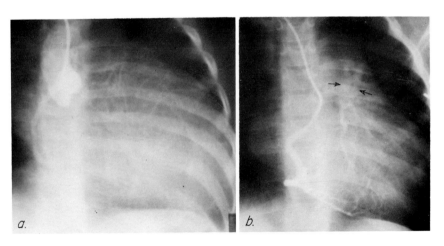

FIG. 63. Characteristic aortographic studies in anomalous origin of the left coronary artery from the pulmonary trunk. *a.* An early phase in which only the right coronary artery is opacified. *b.* The late stage in which collaterals leading to the left coronary system are shown. Slight opacification of pulmonary trunk (between arrows) is also evident.

the pulmonary trunk (Fig. 63b). Left ventriculography demonstrates mitral insufficiency if present.

Angiographic demonstration of collaterals between the two coronary arteries tends to be increasingly apparent with increasing age of patients. Occasionally, injection of contrast material either into the right ventricular cavity or the pulmonary trunk may show opacification of the left anomalously arising coronary artery (107, 115). The diagnostic methods of choice, however, are aortography and left ventriculography.

Hemodynamics

The dynamics in this condition can be best understood if they are related to the pressure and resistance in the pulmonary arterial system (27, 28). During fetal life, the pulmonary arterial pressure equals aortic pressure and the perfusion pressure in the anomalous artery must be assumed to be equal to that in the normally arising right coronary artery. During fetal life one can assume that the pulmonary trunk supplies the coronary flow in a normal fashion. When, after birth, the level of the pulmonary arterial pressure falls, there is a corresponding fall in the perfusion pressure within the left coronary artery (Fig. 53). At this early stage collaterals leading from the normally arising right coronary artery into the left coronary artery may not be well developed, and myocardial ischemia may occur on the basis of inadequate flow into the myocardium of the left ventricle. If the patient survives, the low pressure in the left coronary arterial branches invites the development of collaterals into the left system from the right coronary artery (Fig. 54). Establishment of collateral flow from the right into the left coronary artery may occur in infancy and resembles the situation seen in an arteriovenous communication. The right coronary arterial blood derived from the aorta (oxygenated) is shunted into the pulmonary trunk (unoxygenated) through the anomalous left coronary. Ischemia of the myocardium is a manifestation of inadequate perfusion pressure in the coronary arterial system. After an arteriovenous fistula-like state is established, ischemia occurs in a manner similar to that when both coronary arteries arise from the aorta and one communicates with the cardiac chamber. The different stages of the hemodynamics related to the levels of pressure in the pulmonary arterial system and the development of collateral circulation are shown in the diagram (Fig. 61). The presence of a left-to-right shunt may not be detected when right-sided catheterization is performed.

In children older than one and one-half years, shunts of a significant magnitude have been described (19, 93, 94). It is of interest that in the two adult patients described by Roche (88) and by Baue and associates (9) the left-to-right shunt was not detected on catheterization. On selective aortography, however, a left-to-right shunt was well visualized. In both patients, anginal pain was described and Baue's group called this situation a "coronary steal" syndrome.

Treatment

The conservative treatment of this anomaly is to treat the congestive heart failure. Apart from this conservative treatment, the treatment of anomalous origin of the left coronary artery from the pulmonary artery is surgical (9, 97). In 1949, Gasul and Loeffler (34) proposed an aortic-pulmonary anastomosis to increase pulmonary arterial pressure. This procedure was attempted but was not successful (98). Kittle and associates (53), in 1955, proposed the bending of the pulmonary artery, hoping that increase in the systolic pressure in the pulmonary trunk would improve the flow through the left coronary artery. Surgical methods for increasing collateral circulation, such as pudrage and de-epicardialization, have also been applied. Baisch and Giknis (8) reported on a child who developed constrictive pericarditis after pudrage and abrasion of the pericardium. Ligation of the left coronary artery was suggested by Edwards (28). The purpose of this procedure was to stop the flow to the pulmonary artery and thus allow better perfusion in the left coronary system. This operation is of help only when one can prove that the blood flows from the anomalous left coronary artery into the pulmonary artery.

Mustard (71) removed a segment of the pulmonary artery surrounding the left coronary artery ostium and anastomosed this segment to the left common carotid artery. Although the procedure was completed successfully, ventricular fibrillation developed and the patient died. Apley and associates (6) attempted a similar anastomosis between the left coronary artery and the left subclavian artery. The patient died postoperatively. Bookstein (13) was the first to report a successful anastomosis of the left coronary artery originating in the pulmonary artery to the aorta in 1964. The four-month-old boy, however, died a few hours after operation. In 1966, Cooley and associates (22) reported two cases of successful division of the left coronary artery from the pulmonary trunk and anatomosis to the aorta was accomplished. In one case, he used a Dacron graft, while in the other, he used a segment of autogenous saphenous vein. Both operations were successful and the grafts were functioning well several weeks after the operation. Wesselhoeft and associates (112), reviewing the 26 cases reported in the literature in which the anomalous left coronary artery was ligated at its origin, pointed out that 20 of the patients were infants and six were children (6, 18, 24, 46, 52, 58, 65, 72, 73, 75, 78, 81, 85, 95–98, 104, 107, 113).

The six children survived, but 10 of the 20 infants (50%) succumbed: eight from ventricular fibrillation, one from congestive failure (18), and the other died suddenly (46). This suggests that collaterals between the two coronary arteries progressively enlarge so that the older the patient, the safer is the procedure of interruption of the anomalous artery. If circumstances allow, it would appear ideal to delay operation until the period of infancy is passed.

Anomalous Origin of the Right Coronary Artery from the Pulmonary Artery (Fig. 64 and 65)

The right coronary artery arises from the right pulmonary sinus and follows the usual course of distribution along the right atrioventricular groove. In the case of Jordan and associates (49) the posterior descending artery arose from the left circumflex rather than from the anomalous right coronary artery.

The pulmonary arterial ostium of the right coronary artery has been described as high in these cases, the highest being located 15 mm above the free margin of the pulmonary valve. The right coronary artery is usually described as thin or veinlike on gross examination, although histologically

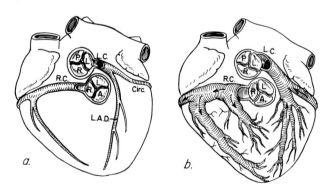

FIG. 64. Anomalous origin of right coronary artery from the pulmonary trunk. *a.* At a stage in which collaterals are not yet well developed. *b.* At a stage in which collaterals between the two coronary systems are highly developed and the coronary arterial vessels have become dilated and tortuous.

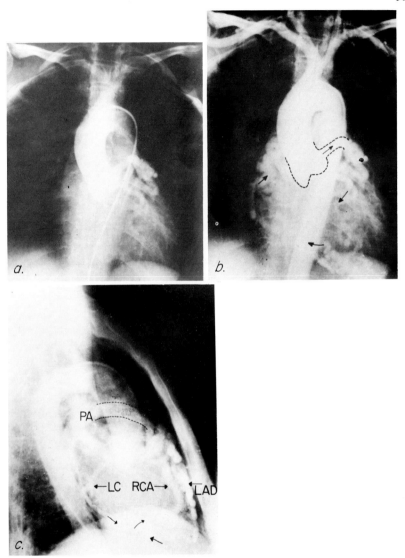

FIG. 65. Aortography in anomalous origin of the right coronary artery from the pulmonary trunk in a 42-year-old woman. *a.* Frontal view of early phase. Only the left coronary artery is opacified. *b.* Late phase. The left coronary artery and the right coronary artery are now opacified. Arrows indicate direction of flow of blood. *c.* Lateral view. The right coronary artery (RCA) is enlarged and opacified. There is also opacification of the pulmonary artery (PA). From a case submitted by Dr. Robert C. Schlant.

the vessel has the basic structure of an artery. Burroughs and associates (16) described a case in which the right coronary artery was of normal thickness. In this case, pulmonary hypertension may be assumed on the basis of the presence of aortopulmonary and ventricular septal defects. In contrast, in the cases in which the right coronary artery is thin, the pulmonary arterial pressure may be considered to have been normal.

In all cases, the left coronary artery has a normal origin and distribution. Evidently this situation is compatible with the metabolic requirements of the myocardium nourished by the right coronary artery, for no clinical or pathologic evidence of ischemia or infarction along the course of the right coronary artery has been described.

No auscultatory or electrocardiographic abnormalities have been described specific to this anomalous origin of the right coronary artery.

Recently antemortem diagnoses by angiocardiography have been reported. The patient described by Ranniger and associates (82) was a six and one-half-year-old girl. A grade IV/VI systolic and a grade II/VI diastolic murmur were present at the apex as well as in the left anterior axillary line at the fifth intercostal space. The electrocardiogram showed evidence of right ventricular hypertrophy and the thoracic roentgenogram showed evidence of mild enlargement of the heart with right atrial and right ventricular dilatation. The pulmonary vasculature was within normal limits. Cardiac catheterization revealed desaturation of the systemic arterial blood (85% saturation), but no left-to-right shunt was conclusively demonstrated. Pulmonary arterial, infundibular and right ventricular pressures were 12/8, 28/5 and 110/6 mm Hg, respectively. A cineangiogram revealed right ventricular infundibular stenosis and a ventricular septal defect with bi-directional shunt. Retrograde aortography revealed a normal site of origin for the left coronary artery, while the right artery was not visualized. The left artery was dilated and tortuous with prominent branches of the anterior descending coronary artery. Multiple small, irregular vessels were observed throughout the entire myocardium associated with filling of a vessel in the position of the right coronary artery. Late films showed the right coronary artery entering the right lateral aspect of the main pulmonary artery. In addition, a patent ductus was present.

Wald and associates (110) have diagnosed two similar cases antemortem by means of aortography. Their second case involving a 17-year-old boy was of special interest in that electrocardiographic changes of ischemia were demonstrated. This patient died suddenly. Pathologic examination showed the left coronary artery arising normally from the left aortic sinus, while the right coronary artery, which was thin and veinlike, arose from the main pulmonary artery several millimeters above the pulmonary valve. The right coronary artery was normal in its distribution and did not show gross communication with the left coronary circulation. The left main coronary artery showed marked intimal thickening with a basophilic fibrocollagenous tissue and was totally obstructed by fresh thrombus. This might have been responsible for the electrocardiographic changes, although the age of the thrombus was not correlated with the time when ischemic changes became evident.

The prognosis in cases in which the right coronary artery originates from the pulmonary trunk appears to be good. Gasul and associates (33), in 1960, stated that surgical correction is not necessary; however, in patients surviving to adulthood, considerable atherosclerosis is present in the left coronary artery, seemingly not basically different from that seen in control cases. This process was probably the cause of death in Pribble's patient (80).

As experience with grafting increases, one might consider in the future grafting the right coronary artery to the aorta. In the case reported by Rowe and Young (90), the patient underwent operation with a preoperative diagnosis of atrial septal defect. Instead, an anomalous right coronary artery was found. The vessel was ligated and the postoperative course was uneventful.

ANOMALOUS ORIGIN OF BOTH CORONARY ARTERIES FROM THE PULMONARY ARTERY (FIG. 66)

In the rare condition in which the entire coronary arterial supply is from the pulmonary trunk, there are usually two coronary arteries, rarely a single coronary artery. Only the condition in which two arteries are present and arise from the pulmonary trunk, is considered in this section. The condition in which there is a single coronary artery and this vessel arises from the pulmonary trunk will be considered in the next section.

In the reported cases of both coronary arteries arising from the pulmonary trunk, the patients have died when less than two weeks of age (5, 11, 37, 39, 47, 60, 87, 101, 103, 114, 116).

Concomitant cardiovascular defects were present in most cases, a patent ductus arteriosus being the most common. Williams and associates (114) reported a case of tetralogy of Fallot. A number of anomalies were found in the case of Grayzel and Tennant (39): tricuspid atresia, two ventricular septal defects, origin of the right pulmonary artery from the

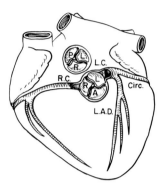

FIG. 66. Anomalous origin of both coronary arteries from the pulmonary trunk.

aorta, and a coronary sinus that emptied into the right and left atria. Gonzalez-Angulo and associates (37) described coarctation of the aorta and a ventricular septal defect. In 1937, Limbourg (60) reported this anomaly in a 10-day-old boy with a patent ductus arteriosus and no other cardiac anomalies. In 1951, Williams and co-workers (114) found this anomaly in a four-day-old girl with tetralogy of Fallot. In 1954, Tedeschi and Helpern (105) described the case of a 13-day-old girl with anomalous origin of both pulmonary arteries and with a patent ductus arteriosus. Schulze and Rodin (101), in 1961, described autopsy findings in a 27-day-old girl. The two coronary arteries arose from the pulmonary artery, the right coronary artery from the region of the right pulmonary sinus, and the left coronary artery from the left pulmonary sinus. The distribution of both coronary arteries was normal. Microscopic examination of the myocardium of the left ventricle revealed areas of interstitial edema with leukocytic infiltration suggestive of early ischemia.

Limbourg (60) and Swann and Werthammer (103) mentioned finding myocardial changes in their cases which were compatible with ischemia. In 1964, Blake and associates (11) described the case of an infant who died 2 hours after birth, in whom both coronary arteries originated from the left pulmonary sinus. No clinical or additional pathologic data were mentioned in this case.

Alexander and Griffith (5), in 1956, described a two-day-old boy in whom both coronary arteries arose from the pulmonary artery. A patent foramen ovale and a patent ductus arteriosus were also present. Schulze and Rodin (101) noted veinlike arteries. Tedeschi and Helpern (105) found thickening of the arterial walls due to an intimal fibrous proliferation and focal edema of the media and adventitia.

Clinically, cyanosis and dyspnea within the first few hours after birth are common and, in part, are related to associated malformations.

Thoracic roentgenography is nonspecific. Enlargement of the cardiac silhouette is variable. The pulmonary vasculature may be increased. Electrocardiographic studies, which were described in only one case (103), showed right axis deviation, right atrial hypertrophy and right ventricular hypertrophy.

If the condition should be diagnosed clinically, treatment may be complicated by the frequently present associated conditions.

Anomalous Origin of a Single Coronary Artery from the Pulmonary Artery (Fig. 67)

In this malformation, the myocardium receives its entire blood supply from a single coronary artery arising from the pulmonary trunk. Only five cases have been described (21, 32, 70, 76, 106). This anomaly had been considered to be incompatible with life for more than a few weeks. Among the reported cases, some patients survived as long as seven years.

The case described by Tow (106) was that of a five-month-old girl whose death was caused by congestive heart failure. Autopsy disclosed persistent truncus arteriosus with both pulmonary arteries arising separately from the posterior aspect of the truncus. No coronary arteries arose from the truncus. A single ostium of the coronary artery was found in the

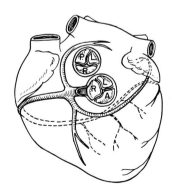

FIG. 67. Single coronary artery arising from pulmonary trunk. A ventricular septal defect was also present. Diagrammatic portrayal of case from ref. 70.

left pulmonary artery just after its origin from the persistent truncus. No ostium was seen for the right coronary artery and the single coronary artery was not traced distally.

The case described by Colmers and Siderides (21) was that of a 33-day-old boy. Autopsy revealed no coronary ostia in the aorta. A single large coronary ostium was present in the left sinus of the pulmonary artery. Just beyond its ostium the single coronary artery divided into the right and left branches. The right coronary artery followed a course between the aorta and the pulmonary artery to reach the right atrioventricular groove. The distal branching of the right and left coronary arteries appeared to be normal. The left ventricle showed massive infarction.

The case described by Feldt and associates (32) was that of a seven-year-old girl who died after surgical closure of a ventricular septal defect. This patient also had a patent ductus arteriosus which was ligated 10 months prior to correction of the septal defect. A holosystolic murmur, grade IV/VI, was heard at the lower left atrial border and an apical mid-diastolic rumble, grade II, without presystolic crescendo was present. A blowing decrescendo diastolic murmur, grade II, was heard in the pulmonic area. The roentgenogram of the thorax showed cardiomegaly with slightly increased pulmonary vasculature. The electrocardiogram showed normal sinus rhythm with a mean manifest electrical axis of the QRS complex of −10 degrees, left atrial hypertrophy, and right ventricular overload. At autopsy, a valvular competent patent foramen ovale was present. The right atrium and tricuspid valve were normal. The ventricular septal defect, measuring 1 cm in diameter, was in the usual position and had been closed completely by a Teflon patch. The free wall of the right ventricle was 1.2 cm thick.

No coronary arteries originated from the aorta whose valve was normal. A single coronary arterial ostium was present in the posterior wall of the pulmonary trunk, 0.5 cm above the level of the tricuspid pulmonary valve (Fig. 68). At its origin from the pulmonary trunk, the single coronary ostium measured 1.5 mm in diameter. The main distribution of the single artery was in the left atrioventricular sulcus in the position of the left circumflex artery. Five millimeters from its origin, the coronary artery gave off two small branches. One was less than 1 mm in diameter and passed posteriorly to the aortic root to reach the right atrioventricular groove; this branch constituted the right coronary artery. The other branch was the anterior descending coronary artery. It descended over the anterior aspect of the heart in the interventricular sulcus, following the

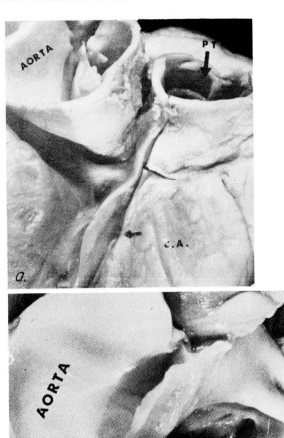

FIG. 68. From the case shown diagrammatically in Fig. 67. Pathologic features of origin of single coronary artery from the pulmonary trunk associated with ventricular septal defect. *a.* Transsected aorta and pulmonary trunk (PT). Only a single coronary artery is present (C.A.). This arises from the pulmonary trunk. Its epicardial course along the right aspect of the heart is shown. *b.* Interior of base of left ventricle and ascending aorta. An impression (D) is present in the wall of the right aortic sinus but no coronary ostia are present in the aorta. A ventricular septal defect (VSD) is present.

usual course for the anterior descending artery. The diameter of the left anterior descending coronary artery was less than 1 mm.

Ogden's patient (76) was a six-day-old girl who, on the third day of life, was found to have a holosystolic murmur, grade III/VI. An electrocardiogram showed evidence of right ventricular hypertrophy, while the thoracic roentgenogram revealed cardiomegaly with slightly increased pulmonary vasculature. The child died at the age of six days. Autopsy revealed a widely patent ductus arteriosus and a widely patent foramen ovale. The ostium of a large single coronary artery was found in the left pulmonary sinus. This gave rise to a vessel which immediately divided into right and left branches. The left branch subsequently divided into the circumflex and anterior descending branches. The right branch of the single coronary artery coursed between the pulmonary artery and the aorta and then assumed a normal course for the right coronary artery in the right atrioventricular groove. Microscopic examination of the myocardium was unremarkable. No areas of infarction were noted.

In the case described by Monselise and associates (70), a ventricular septal defect and pulmonary hypertension were present. Cyanosis with moderate dyspnea was noted immediately after birth. On examination, a heave of both ventricles was palpable, there were no thrills, and at the apex area, the first sound was accentuated. In the left fourth intercostal space, a diastolic flow murmur and a pansystolic murmur were audible. The latter radiated to the base of the heart and to the neck. The electrocardiogram showed a mean manifest electrical axis of the QRS complex in the frontal plane of + 140 degrees and signs of right and left ventricular hypertrophy. Thoracic roentgenograms showed cardiomegaly and increased pulmonary vasculature. The child died at the age of one year from an intercurrent infection. At autopsy, the following findings were observed: The heart weighed 110 g. A network of prominent coronary arteries covered its surface. The right atrium was enlarged, and a probe-patent foramen was present. The right ventricle was hypertrophied. Its wall measured 9 mm in thickness. A ventricular septal defect measuring 8 mm in diameter was present. A single coronary artery was present that arose from the right sinus of the pulmonary valve. Its orifice measured 2 mm in diameter (Fig. 68).

About 4 mm from its origin, the single coronary artery trifurcated. The main branch proceeded into the right atrioventricular sulcus. A second branch was short and, in turn, divided into anterior descending and left circumflex branches. The third branch was a wide atrial artery (Fig. 67).

The left ventricle did not show any signs of ischemic change. The papillary muscles were normal. Histologically, the coronary arteries showed moderate changes in the intima and a normal media.

The lungs were dark, heavy and edematous and the lower lobes were friable due to bronchopneumonia. The liver and the spleen were both congested. The other organs were normal.

REFERENCES

1. ABBOTT ME. Anomalous origin from the pulmonary arteries, in: Osler W (Ed), "Osler's modern medicine, its theories and practice." Philadelphia, Lea and Febiger, v 4, 1908, p 420.
2. ABRIKOSSOFF A. Aneurysma des linken Herzventrikels mit abnormer Abgangsstelle der linken Koronararterie von der Pulmonalis bei einem fünfmonatlichen Kinde. *Virchows Arch [Pathol Anal]* **203**: 413, 1911.
3. AGUSTSSON MH, GASUL BM, FELL EH, GRAETTINGER JS, BICOFF JP and WATERMAN DF. Anomalous origin of left coronary artery from pulmonary artery: Diagnosis and treatment of infantile and adult types. *JAMA* **180**: 15, 1962.
4. AGUSTSSON MH, GASUL BM and LUNDQUIST R. Anomalous origin of the left coronary artery from the pulmonary artery (adult type). A case report. *Pediatrics* **29**: 274, 1962.
5. ALEXANDER RW and GRIFFITH GC. Anomalies of the coronary arteries and their clinical significance. *Circulation* **14**: 800, 1956.
6. APLEY J, HORTON RE and WILSON MG. Possible role of surgery in the treatment of anomalous left coronary artery. *Thorax* **12**: 28, 1957.
7. ARMER RM, SHUMACKER HB JR, LURIE PR and FISCH C. Origin of the left coronary artery from the pulmonary artery without collateral circulation: Report of a case with a suggested surgical correction. *Pediatrics* **32**: 588, 1963.
8. BAISCH BF and GIKNIS FL. Rare anomalies of coronary circulation amenable to surgical correction. Left coronary to pulmonary artery fistula and supernumerary coronary artery. *Ann Thorac Surg* **1**: 170, 1965.
9. BAUE AE, BAUM S, BLAKEMORE WS and ZINSSER HF. A later stage of anomalous coronary circulation with origin of the left coronary artery from the pulmonary artery. Coronary artery steal. *Circulation* **36**: 878, 1967.
10. BAYLISS JH and CAMPBELL M. An unusual cause for a continuous murmur. *Guys Hosp Rep* **101**: 174, 1952.
11. BLAKE HA, MANION WC, MATTINGLY TW and BAROLDI G. Coronary artery anomalies. *Circulation* **30**: 927, 1964.
12. BLAND EF, WHITE PD and GARLAND J. Congenital anomalies of the coronary arteries: Report of an unusual case associated with cardiac hypertrophy. *Am Heart J* **8**: 787, 1933.
13. BOOKSTEIN JJ. Aberrant left coronary artery. *Am J Roentgenol Radium Ther Nucl Med* **91**: 515, 1964.
14. BROOKS H ST J. Two cases of an abnormal coronary artery of the heart arising from the pulmonary artery: With some remarks upon the effect of this anomaly in producing cirsoid dilatation of the vessels. *J Anat Physiol* **20**: 26, 1886.
15. BURCHELL HB and BROWN AL JR. Anomalous origin of coronary artery from pulmonary artery masquerading as mitral insufficiency. *Am Heart J* **63**: 388, 1962.
16. BURROUGHS JT, SCHMUTZER KJ, LINDER F and NEUHAUS G. Anomalous origin of the right coronary artery with aortico-pulmonary window and ventricular septal defect. *J Cardiovasc Surg* **3**: 142, 1962.

17. CARRINGTON G and KRUMBHAAR EB. So-called idiopathic cardiac hypertrophy in infancy. *Am J Dis Child* **27**: 449, 1924.
18. CASE RB, MORROW AG, STAINSBY W and NESTOR JO. Anomalous origin of the left coronary artery: The physiologic defect and suggested surgical treatment. *Circulation* **17**: 1062, 1958.
19. COATES JR, TIMMIS HH and SCOTT LP III. Anomalous left coronary artery, transitional stage. *Am J Cardiol* **17**: 286, 1966.
20. COHEN H and SIEW S. Aberrant left coronary artery: Report of a case and review of the literature. *Circulation* **20**: 918, 1959.
21. COLMERS RA and SIDERIDES CI. Anomalous origin of both coronary arteries from the pulmonary trunk. Myocardial infarction in otherwise normal heart. *Am J Cardiol* **12**: 263, 1963.
22. COOLEY DA, HALLMAN GL and BLOODWELL RD. Definitive surgical treatment of anomalous origin of left coronary artery from pulmonary artery: Indications and results. *J Thorac Cardiovasc Surg* **52**: 798, 1966.
23. CRONK ES, SINCLAIR JG and RIGDON RH. An anomalous coronary artery arising from the pulmonary artery. *Am Heart J* **42**: 906, 1951.
24. CUMMING GR and FERGUSON CC. Anomalous origin of the left coronary artery from the pulmonary artery, functioning as a coronary arteriovenous fistula. *Am Heart J* **64**: 690, 1962.
25. DIETRICH W. Ursprung der vorderen Kranzarterie aus der Lungenschlagader mit ungewöhnlichen Veränderungen des Herzmuskels und der Gefässwände. *Virchows Arch [Pathol Anat]* **303**: 436, 1939.
26. EDWARDS JE. Functional pathology of congenital cardiac disease. *Pediatr Clin North Am* **1**: 13, 1954.
27. EDWARDS JE. Anomalous coronary arteries with special reference to arterio-venous-like communications. *Circulation* **17**: 1001, 1958.
28. EDWARDS JE. The direction of blood flow in coronary arteries arising from the pulmonary trunk. *Circulation* **29**: 163, 1964.
29. EIDLOW S and MACKENZIE ER. Anomalous origin of the left coronary artery from the pulmonary artery: Report of a case diagnosed clinically and confirmed by necropsy. *Am Heart J* **32**: 243, 1946.
30. ESTES EH JR, DALTON FM, ENTMAN ML, DIXON HB II and HACKEL DB. The anatomy and blood supply of the papillary muscles of the left ventricle. *Am Heart J* **71**: 356, 1966.
31. ESTES EH JR, ENTMAN ML, DIXON HB II and HACKEL DB. The vascular supply of the left ventricular wall: Anatomic observations, plus a hypothesis regarding acute events in coronary artery disease. *Am Heart J* **71**: 58, 1966.
32. FELDT RH, ONGLEY PA and TITUS JL. Total coronary arterial circulation from pulmonary artery with survival to age seven: report of case. *Mayo Clin Proc* **40**: 539, 1965.
33. GASUL BM, ARCILLA RA, FELL EH, LYNFIELD J, BICOFF JP and LUAN LL. Congenital coronary arteriovenous fistula. Clinical, phonocardiographic, angiocardiographic and hemodynamic studies in five patients. *Pediatrics* **25**: 531, 1960.
34. GASUL BM and LOEFFLER E. Anomalous origin of the left coronary artery from the pulmonary artery (Bland-White-Garland syndrome). Report of 4 cases. *Pediatrics* **4**: 498, 1949.
35. GEORGE JM and KNOWLAN DM. Anomalous origin of the left coronary artery from the pulmonary artery in an adult. *N Engl J Med* **261**: 993, 1959.
36. GOLDBERGER E. Angiocardiographic diagnosis of an anomalous left coronary artery originating from the pulmonary artery: Progress notes in cardiology. *Am J Cardiol* **6**: 694, 1960.
37. GONZALEZ-ANGULO A, REYES HA and WALLACE SA. Anomalies of the origin of coronary arteries. Special reference to single coronary artery. *Angiology* **17**: 96, 1966.
38. GOULEY BA. Anomalous left coronary artery arising from the pulmonary artery (adult type). *Am Heart J* **40**: 630, 1950.

39. GRAYZEL DM and TENNANT R. Congenital atresia of the tricuspid orifice and anomalous origins of the coronary arteries from the pulmonary artery. *Am J Pathol* **10**: 791, 1934.
40. HALLMAN GL, COOLEY DA and SINGER DB. Congenital anomalies of the coronary arteries: Anatomy, pathology and surgical treatment. *Surgery* **59**: 133, 1966.
41. HARTENSTEIN H and FREEMAN DJ. Origin of left coronary artery from pulmonary artery. *Am J Dis Child* **83**: 774, 1952.
42. HEATH D and EDWARDS JE. The pathology of hypertensive pulmonary vascular disease: A description of six grades of structural changes in the pulmonary arteries with special reference to congenital cardiac septal defects. *Circulation* **18**: 533, 1958.
43. HEITZMANN O. Drei seltene Fälle von Herzmissbildung. Virchows Arch [*Pathol Anat*] **223**: 57, 1917.
44. HELPERN MG. Cited by Kaunitz PE (51).
45. HORLICK L, MERRIMAN JE and ROBINSON LN. A case of mitral insufficiency following myocardial infarction with rupture of papillary muscle: Improvement following reattachment of the papillary muscle and plication of the mitral valve. *Can Med Assoc J* **94**: 192, 1966.
46. HUNG W and WALSH BJ. Anomalous left coronary artery arising from the pulmonary artery: Report of a case diagnosed clinically and operated upon, with autopsy findings. *Clin Proc Child Hosp DC* **16**: 228, 1960.
47. JAMES TN. Anatomy of the coronary arteries. New York, Paul B Hoebe, 1961.
48. JAMESON AG, ELLIS K and LEVINE OR. Anomalous left coronary artery arising from pulmonary artery. *Br Heart J* **25**: 251, 1963.
49. JORDAN RA, DRY TJ and EDWARDS JE. Anomalous origin of the right coronary artery from the pulmonary trunk. *Proc Mayo Clin* **25**: 673, 1950.
50. JURISHICA AJ. Anomalous left coronary artery: Adult type. *Am Heart J* **54**: 429, 1957.
51. KAUNITZ PE. Origin of the left coronary artery from the pulmonary artery: Review of the literature and a report of 2 cases. *Am Heart J* **33**: 182, 1947.
52. KEITH JD. The anomalous origin of the left coronary artery from the pulmonary artery. *Br Heart J* **21**: 149, 1959.
53. KITTLE CF, DIEHL AM and HEILBRUNN A. Anomalous left coronary artery arising from the pulmonary artery: Report of a case and surgical consideration. *J Pediatr* **47**: 198, 1955.
54. KOCKEL H. Eigenartige Kranzschlagadermissbildungen. *Beitr Pathol Anat* **94**: 220, 1934.
55. KUZMAN WJ, YUSKIS AS and CARMICHAEL DB. Anomalous left coronary artery arising from the pulmonary artery. *Am Heart J* **57**: 36, 1959.
56. LAMBERT EC, SHUMWAY CN and TERPLAN K. Clinical diagnosis of endocardial fibrosis: Analysis of literature with report of 4 new cases. *Pediatrics* **11**: 255, 1953.
57. LAMPE CFJ and VERHEUGT APM. Anomalous left coronary artery. Adult type. *Am Heart J* **59**: 769, 1960.
58. LIEBMAN J, HELLERSTEIN HK, ANKENEY JL and TUCKER A. The problem of the anomalous left coronary artery arising from the pulmonary artery in older children: Report of three cases. *N Engl J Med* **269**: 486, 1963.
59. LIKAR I, CRILEY JM and LEWIS KB. Anomalous left coronary artery arising from the pulmonary artery in an adult: A review of the therapeutic problem. *Circulation* **33**: 727, 1966.
60. LIMBOURG M. Über den Ursprung der Kranzarterien des Herzens aus der Arteria pulmonalis. *Beitr Pathol Anat* **100**: 191, 1937.
61. LINTERMANS JP, KAPLAN EL, MORGAN BC, BAUM D and GUNTHEROTH WG. Infarction patterns in endocardial fibroelastosis. *Circulation* **33**: 202, 1966.

62. LOSEKOOT G, RENAUD EJ, MEYNE NG and VAN DAM RT. Anomalous left coronary artery arising from the pulmonary artery. A report on two cases with successful surgical therapy. *Br Heart J* **28**: 646, 1966.

63. MCKINLEY HI, ANDREWS J and NEILL CA. Left coronary artery from the pulmonary artery: Three cases, one with cardiac tamponade. *Pediatrics* **8**: 828, 1951.

64. MASEL L. Tetralogy of Fallot with origin of the left coronary artery from the right pulmonary artery. *Med J Aust* **1**: 213, 1960.

65. MASSIH NA, LAWLER J and VERMILLION M. Myocardial ischemia after ligation of an anomalous left coronary artery arising from the pulmonary artery. *N Engl J Med* **269**: 483, 1963.

66. MICHAUD P, FROMENT R, VIARD H, GRAVIER J and VERNEY RN. Coronary-right ventricular fistulas: Apropos of 3 operated cases. *Arch Mal Coeur* **56**: 143, 1963.

67. MILLER RD, BURCHELL HB and EDWARDS JE. Myocardial infarction with and without acute coronary occlusion: Pathologic study. *Arch Intern Med* **88**: 597, 1951.

68. MOLLER JH, LUCAS RV JR, ADAMS P JR, ANDERSON RC, JORGENS J and EDWARDS JE. Endocardial fibroelastosis: A clinical and anatomic study of 47 patients with emphasis on its relationship to mitral insufficiency. *Circulation* **30**: 759, 1964.

69. MÖNCKEBERG JG. Über eine seltene Anomalie des Koronararterienabgangs. *Zbl Herz Gefässkr* **6**: 441, 1914.

70. MONSELISE MB, VLODAVER Z and NEUFELD HN. Single coronary artery; origin from the pulmonary trunk in association with ventricular septal defect. *Chest* **58**: 613, 1970.

71. MUSTARD A. Cited by Sabiston DC Jr (95). Also Discussion (96).

72. NADAS AS. "Pediatric cardiology," 2nd edn. Philadelphia, WB Saunders, 1963, p 261.

73. NADAS AS, GAMBOA R and HUGENHOLTZ PG. Anomalous left coronary artery originating from the pulmonary artery: Report of two surgically treated cases with a proposal of hemodynamic and therapeutic classification. *Circulation* **29**: 167, 1964.

74. NORA JJ, MCNAMARA DG, HALLMAN GL, SUMMERVILLE RJ and COOLEY DA. Medical and surgical management of anomalous origin of left coronary artery from the pulmonary artery. *Pediatrics* **42**: 405, 1968.

75. NOREN GR, RAGHIB G, MOLLER JH, AMPLATZ K, ADAMS P JR and EDWARDS JE. Anomalous origin of the left coronary artery from the pulmonary trunk with special reference to the occurrence of mitral insufficiency. *Circulation* **30**: 171, 1964.

76. OGDEN JA. Origin of a single coronary artery from the pulmonary artery. *Am Heart J* **78**: 251, 1969.

77. ORSOS F. Über die Rolle der Coronargefässe beim Altern des Herzens. *Beitr Pathol Anat* **106**: 1, 1942.

78. PAUL RN and ROBBINS SG. Surgical treatment proposed for either endocardial fibroelastosis or anomalous left coronary artery. *Circulation* **16**: 147, 1955.

79. PHILLIPS JH, BURCH GE and DE PASQUALE NP. The syndrome of papillary muscle dysfunction: Its clinical recognition. *Ann Intern Med* **59**: 508, 1963.

80. PRIBBLE RH. Anatomic variations of the coronary arteries and their clinical significance. The third reported case of an unusual anomaly. *J Indiana Med Ass* **54**: 329, 1961.

81. PURI PS, ROWE RD and NEILL CA. Varying vectorcardiographic patterns in anomalous left coronary artery arising from pulmonary artery. *Am Heart J* **71**: 616, 1966.

82. RANNIGER K, THILENIUS OG and CASSELS DE. Angiographic diagnosis of an anomalous right coronary artery arising from the pulmonary artery. *Radiology* **88**: 29, 1967.

83. RAO BNS, LUCAS RV JR and EDWARDS JE. Anomalous origin of the left coronary artery from the right pulmonary artery associated with ventricular septal defect. *Chest* **59**: 616, 1970.

84. RECAVARREN S and ARIAS-STELLA J. Growth and development of the ventricular myocardium from birth to adult life. *Br Heart J* **26**: 187, 1964.

85. REED WA and KITTLE CF. Congenital coronary artery fistula. *Arch Surg* **93**: 772, 1966.

86. REINER L, MOLNAR J, JIMENEZ FA and FREUDENTHAL RR. Interarterial coronary anastomoses in neonates. *Arch Pathol* **71**: 103, 1961.

87. ROBERTS JT and LOUBE SD. Congenital single coronary artery in man. Report of nine new cases, one having thrombosis with right ventricular and atrial (auricular) infarction. *Am Heart J* **34**: 188, 1947.

88. ROCHE AHG. Anomalous origin of the left coronary artery from the pulmonary artery in the adult. Report of uneventful ligation in two cases. *Am J Cardiol* **20**: 561, 1967.

89. ROTTER W. Über den abnormen Abgang der linken Herzkranzarterie aus der Lungenschlagader. *Zbl Allg Pathol Anat* **89**: 160, 1952.

90. ROWE GG and YOUNG WP. Anomalous origin of the coronary arteries with special reference to surgical treatment. *J Thorac Cardiovasc Surg* **39**: 777, 1960.

91. RUBBERDT H. Abnormer Abgang der linken Kranzarterie aus der Lungenschlagader. *Beitr Pathol Anat* **98**: 571, 1937.

92. RUDDOCK JC and STEHLY CC. Anomalous origin of left coronary artery: Case report. *US Nav Med Bull* **41**: 175, 1943.

93. RUDOLPH AM. The effects of postnatal circulatory adjustments in congenital heart disease. *Pediatrics* **36**: 763, 1965.

94. RUDOLPH AM, GOOTMAN NL, KAPLAN N and ROHMAN M. Anomalous left coronary artery arising from the pulmonary artery with large left-to-right shunt in infancy. *J Pediatr* **63**: 543, 1963.

95. SABISTON DC JR. Direct surgical management of congenital and acquired lesions of the coronary circulation. *Progr Cardiovasc Dis* **6**: 299, 1963.

96. SABISTON DC JR, NEILL CA and TAUSSIG HB. The direction of blood flow in anomalous left coronary artery arising from the pulmonary artery. *Circulation* **22**: 591, 1960.

97. SABISTON DC JR, PELARGONIO S and TAUSSIG HB. Myocardial infarction in infancy: The surgical management of a complication of congenital origin of the left coronary artery from the pulmonary artery. *J Thorac Cardiovasc Surg* **40**: 321, 1960.

98. SABISTON DC JR, ROSS RS, CRILEY JM. GAERTNER RA, NEILL CA and TAUSSIG HB. Surgical management of congenital lesions of the coronary circulation. *Ann Surg* **157**: 908, 1963.

99. SANES S and KENNY FE. Anomalous origin of left coronary artery from pulmonary artery: with myocardial fibrosis of letf ventricle and partial aneurysm at the apex. *Am J Dis Child* **48**: 113, 1934.

100. SCHLEY J. Abnormer Ursprung der rechten Kranzarterie aus der Pulmonalis bei einem 61-jährigen Mann. *Frankfurt Z Path* **32**: 1, 1925.

101. SCHULZE WB and RODIN AE. Anomalous origin of both coronary arteries. Report of a case with discussion of teratogenetic theories. *Arch Pathol* **72**: 36, 1961.

102. SCHWARTZ RP and ROBICSEK F. An unusual anomaly of the coronary system: origin of the anterior (descending) interventricular artery from the pulmonary trunk. *J Pediatr* **78**: 123, 1971.

103. SWANN WC and WERTHAMMER S. Aberrant coronary arteries: Experiences in diagnosis with report of three cases. *Ann Intern Med* **42**: 873, 1955.

104. TALNER NS, HALLORAN KH, MAHDAVY M, GARDNER TH and HIPONA F. Anomalous origin of the left coronary artery from the pulmonary artery: A clinical spectrum. *Am J Cardiol* **15**: 689, 1965.

105. TEDESCHI CG and HELPERN MM. Heterotopic origin of both coronary arteries from the pulmonary artery: Review of literature and report of a case not complicated by associated defects. *Pediatrics* **14**: 53, 1954.
106. TOW A. Cor biloculare with truncus arteriosus and endocarditis. *Am J Dis Child* **42**: 1413, 1931.
107. USMAN A, FERNANDEZ B, URICCHIO JF and NICHOLS HT. Aberrant origin of left coronary artery combined with mitral regurgitation in an adult. *Am J Cardiol* **8**: 130, 1961.
108. VAN DER HAUWAERT LG, STALPAERT GL and VERHAEGHE L. Anomalous origin of the left coronary artery from the pulmonary artery: A therapeutic problem. *Am Heart J* **69**: 538, 1965.
109. VESTERMARK S. Anomalous origin of left coronary artery from pulmonary trunk. *Acta Paediatr Scand* **54**: 387, 1965.
110. WALD S, STONECIPHER K, BALDWIN BJ and NUTTER DO. Anomalous origin of the right coronary artery from the pulmonary artery. *Am J Cardiol* **27**: 677, 1971.
111. WATSON H. "Pediatric cardiology." St. Louis, CB Mosby, 1950.
112. WESSELHOEFT H, FAWCETT JS and JOHNSON AL. Anomalous origin of the left coronary artery from the pulmonary trunk. Its clinical spectrum, pathology, and pathophysiology, based on a review of 140 cases with seven further cases. *Circulation* **38**: 403, 1968.
113. WILDER RJ and PERLMAN A. Roentgenographic demonstration of anomalous left coronary artery arising from the pulmonary artery. *Am J Roentgenol Radium Ther Nucl Med* **91**: 511, 1964.
114. WILLIAMS JW, JOHNSON WS and BOULWARE JR JR. Case of tetralogy of Fallot with both coronary arteries arising from pulmonary artery. *J Fla Med Assoc* **37**: 561, 1951.
115. WUTHRICH R. Über den Abgang der Arteria coronaria sinistra aus des Arteria pulmonalis: Zugleich ein Beitrag zum Problem des plötzlichen Todes. *Cardiologia* **18**: 193, 1951.
116. ZUMBO O, FANI K, JARMOLYCH J and DAOUD AS. Coronary atherosclerosis and myocardial infarction in hearts with anomalous coronary arteries. *Lab Invest* **14**: 571, 1965.

CHAPTER IX

PATTERNS OF ORIGIN AND DISTRIBUTION OF CORONARY ARTERIES IN TRANSPOSITION COMPLEXES AND TETRALOGY OF FALLOT

Situs solitus (Fig. 69)
Situs inversus
Complete transposition of the great vessels
Corrected transposition of the great vessels
Right ventricular aorta and biventricular pulmonary trunk
Common ventricle with transposition of the great vessels
Origin of both great vessels from the right ventricle (double-outlet right ventricle)
Tetralogy of Fallot
Persistent truncus arteriosus
Angiocardiographic evaluation in transposition of the great vessels

The differential diagnosis of the various transposition complexes is often difficult even though complete clinical, hemodynamic and angiocardiographic data are available. The diagnosis may remain uncertain even at autopsy, especially in cases complicated by dextrocardia, levoversion or a common ventricle.

Although the coronary arterial distributions in the transposition complexes have been studied extensively from the anatomicropathologic point of view, the usefulness of the precise information so attained, concerning the usual or characteristic patterns of these arteries in the presence of each of the various transposition complexes, has not been sufficiently emphasized as a clinical diagnostic tool. This background information used in association with data on the pattern of the coronary arteries as determined by angiocardiography in such cases may give important clues to the diagnosis.

This chapter, therefore, will concern itself with variations in origin and distribution of the coronary arteries in various transposition complexes, including complete transposition, corrected transposition, right ventricular aorta and biventricular pulmonary trunk, single ventricle with transposition, double outlet-right ventricle and tetralogy of Fallot.

The coverage will be both anatomic and angiocardiographic. For this reason, it is appropriate first to define the angiographic characteristics of the aortic sinuses and coronary arteries in the normal (situs solitus) and inverted (situs inversus) positions and in isolated dextrocardia.

SITUS SOLITUS (FIG. 69)

The three pouchlike dilatations of aortic origin are variously called "sinuses of Valsalva" or "aortic sinuses." We recognize the right aortic sinus (RAS), left aortic sinus (LAS), and posterior (noncoronary) aortic sinus (PAS). This terminology may be confusing as it does not correspond to the true topographic location of the sinuses in the heart *in situ* or as delineated by angiocardiography. Thus, in the frontal projection, the PAS and not the RAS is the one located toward the right and most caudally; the LAS is the one farthest to the left and cranially positioned, while the RAS, so called because the right coronary artery originates from it, is actually midway between right and left, lying between the PAS and the LAS. In the lateral projection, the RAS is the most ventrally located; the LAS is the most dorsally and cranially situated, while the PAS projects between the other two sinuses and is the one most caudally situated. The plane of the aortic valve in the frontal projection is oblique and its right

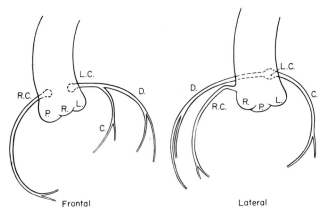

Frontal   Lateral

FIG. 69. Diagrammatic portrayal of angiographic appearances of main coronary arteries in frontal and lateral projections during aortography. C. = left circumflex artery; D. = anterior descending artery.

aspect is lower than its left. In the lateral projection, the tendency toward obliquity of the valve, though present, is less prominent. It is important to realize that the above-mentioned relationships are not significantly influenced by rotation of the heart from extracardiac or intracardiac causes.

Normally, the left coronary artery (LCA) arises from the LAS and courses laterally and ventrally behind the root of the pulmonary trunk (Fig. 69). It divides early into two main branches, the anterior descending one which courses distally in the anterior interventricular sulcus, and the circumflex branch which courses dorsally in the left atrioventricular sulcus.

The right coronary artery (RCA) originates from the RAS and enters the right atrioventricular sulcus. Proximal to the right margin of the heart, the RCA gives off its marginal branch. The parent vessel continues in the right atrioventricular sulcus to the level of the posterior interventricular sulcus. At this point, it turns abruptly toward the apex of the heart and courses in the posterior interventricular sulcus as the posterior descending artery.

When complete visualization of the coronary arteries is achieved angiographically, differentiation of the right from the left coronary artery is no problem. In newborns or infants with severe congenital heart disease or when no special attempts are made to visualize the coronary arteries selectively, this differentiation may however be difficult.

Situs Inversus

In the absence of other anomalies, the feature of situs inversus is that left and right are interchanged from those in situs solitus. Anteroposterior relationships are not disturbed.

Complete Transposition of the Great Vessels

As used here, the term "complete transposition" refers to that condition in which the cardiac chambers are normally formed and oriented, while the aorta arises from the right ventricle and the pulmonary trunk arises from the left ventricle (Fig. 70).

Several pathologic studies have indicated that variations in origin and distribution of the coronary arteries are frequent in transposition of the great vessels (3, 14, 16). These variations bear some relationship to the orientation of the aorta to the pulmonary artery as shown by Elliott and associates (3).

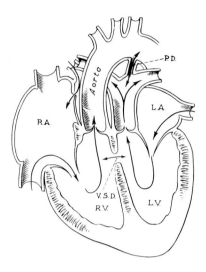

FIG. 70. Complete transposition of great vessels. Diagrammatic portrayal of basic anatomic arrangement. Shown are a ventricular septal defect (V.S.D.) and a patent ductus arteriosus (P.D.). These associated conditions are not universally present in complete transposition.

These authors reported anatomic details in 60 cases of this condition from our laboratories and identified three possible patterns of relationship between the ascending aorta and pulmonary trunk as follows:

In *Type I* (oblique relationship; 39 cases), the aorta was situated obliquely with respect to the pulmonary trunk. Lying toward the right, the aorta was more anterior than the latter vessel. The left side of the ascending aorta lay anterior to the right side of the pulmonary trunk (Fig. 71). In *Type II* (side-to-side relationship; 19 cases), the ascending aorta was situated to the right of the pulmonary trunk (Fig. 71). In *Type III* (anteroposterior relationship; two cases), the ascending aorta lay directly posterior to the pulmonary trunk.

Among the 60 cases, essentially two coronary arterial patterns were observed. The first and more common was seen in 40 of the 60 cases. In these, the pattern of origin and course of the coronary arteries approached that found normally. The left coronary artery gave rise to the anterior descending and the left circumflex branches (Fig. 71). In contrast to the normal pattern, however, the stem of the left coronary artery and the left circumflex coronary artery passed anterior to the pulmonary trunk rather than posterior to it. Furthermore, the right coronary artery

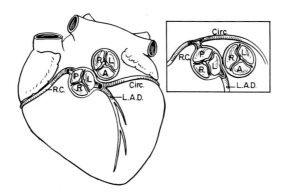

FIG. 71. Complete transposition of great vessels showing the common patterns of coronary arterial origin and distribution in two types of relationship between the great vessels. In the main body of the figure, an oblique relationship exists between the great vessels. The left circumflex artery arises from the left coronary artery. Inset: A side-to-side relationship between the great vessels is shown, wherein the origin of the circumflex artery is commonly from the right coronary artery.

arose above the posterior aortic sinus. From this position, it entered the right atrioventricular sulcus and followed a normal course, frequently anastomosing with the left circumflex branch on the posterior aspect of the heart near the posterior interventricular sulcus.

The second and less common pattern was observed in 20 of the 60 cases. In this, the anterior descending coronary artery arose from the left aortic sinus while the left circumflex coronary artery arose as a branch of the right coronary artery (Fig. 71). The latter vessel, in turn, arose above the posterior aortic sinus.

Illustrated in Fig. 71 are the two basic patterns of coronary arterial origin given in Fig. 69, along with the variations that occurred. From these illustrations, it is evident that the pattern of coronary arterial origin in which the left circumflex and anterior descending arteries have a common stem occurs most often when the great vessels show a Type I (oblique) relationship. When the circumflex coronary artery arises as a branch of the right coronary artery, the prevailing tendency is for the great vessels to manifest a Type II (side-to-side) relationship.

Certain variations from the prevailing coronary arterial pattern were observed in five of the 39 cases with the Type I (oblique) relationship of great vessels (Fig. 72). In one case, two anterior descending coronary arteries were present (Fig. 72c). In two cases, the left coronary artery

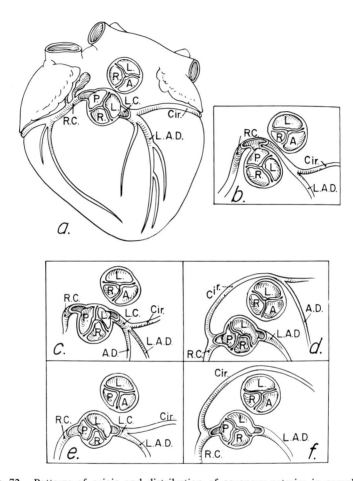

FIG. 72. Patterns of origin and distribution of coronary arteries in complete transposition associated with an oblique relationship between the aorta and the pulmonary
trunk. *a.* The most common pattern. The left coronary artery arises from the left
aortic sinus and branches into its circumflex and anterior descending branches. The
right coronary artery arises from the posterior aortic sinus, while the noncoronary
sinus (R.) is anterior. Variations from this pattern are shown in the insets *b* to *f*.
b. A single coronary artery which branches into the left and right coronary arteries;
the left coronary artery passes anterior to the pulmonary trunk. *c.* Origin of the
left coronary artery as in *a*, but there are two anterior descending branches (A.D.
and L.A.D.). *d.* Origin of the circumflex coronary artery from the right. The
anterior descending coronary artery arises from the left aortic sinus. A second
and smaller anterior descending coronary artery (A.D.) arises from the circumflex
artery after it has coursed behind the pulmonary trunk. *e.* Same pattern as in *a*.
f. Origin of the left circumflex coronary artery from the right coronary artery.
The anterior descending artery arises independently from the left aortic sinus.

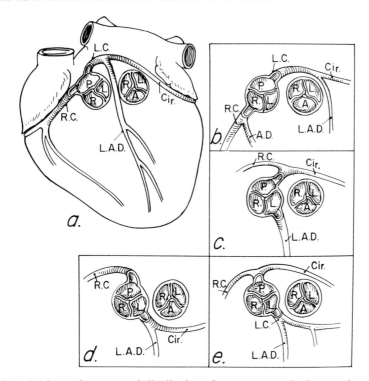

FIG. 73. Origins and patterns of distribution of coronary arteries in complete transposition associated with side-by-side relationship of the great vessels. *a.* One of the less common types in which both the left and right coronary arteries arise from the same (posterior) aortic sinus. *b.* An unusual picture in which the right coronary artery arises from the anterior aortic sinus (R.) and gives rise to the main anterior descending coronary artery. The left coronary artery arises from the posterior aortic sinus (P.) and branches into the circumflex and a smaller anterior descending coronary artery. *c.* The most common pattern when the great vessels lie side-by-side. This is characterized by a common stem of origin for the left circumflex and the right coronary arteries. The anterior descending artery arises directly from the aorta. *d.* The two coronary arteries arise independently from the aorta, while the circumflex coronary artery crosses anterior to the pulmonary trunk. *e.* Origin of the right and left coronary arteries directly from the aorta. One circumflex artery arises from the right coronary artery, another from the left coronary artery.

gave off a large branch from its right side. This branch supplied the base of the right ventricle (Fig. 72*b*). In one case, there was a diverticulum along the left aspect of the right coronary artery; in another, a single coronary artery branched into the right and left coronary arteries (Fig. 72*a*).

In four of the 19 cases with the Type II (side-to-side) relationship of great vessels, certain variations were observed also (Fig. 73). In two cases, two circumflex and two anterior descending coronary arteries were present. In one case, both coronary arteries arose above the posterior sinus, and in another case, the right coronary artery arose above the right aortic sinus (Fig. 73a, inset).

CORRECTED TRANSPOSITION OF THE GREAT VESSELS

Corrected transposition is an established entity in which two ventricles and two atrioventricular valves are present and, except for associated anomalies (that is, ventricular septal defect), the heart could function normally (Fig. 74).

Corrected transposition may be associated either with situs solitus or situs inversus. In situs solitus the left-sided ventricle (that is, the arterial ventricle) is the anatomic right ventricle in inverted orientation and the right-sided ventricle (that is, the venous ventricle) is the anatomic left ventricle (Fig. 74). The aorta is situated at the left basal aspect of the heart and arises from the infundibulum of the left-sided arterial ventricle. The pulmonary trunk arises posteriorly from the venous ventricle and to the right of the transposed ascending aorta.

Two types of relationship are recognized between the aorta and the pulmonary trunk in corrected transposition. In each, the ascending aorta arises from the left ventrobasal aspect of the heart. In one type (more

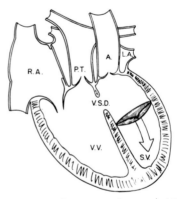

FIG. 74. Basic anatomic arrangement in corrected transposition which is characterized by inversion of the ventricles and atrioventricular valves, as well as transposition and inversion of the great vessels. The basic connections are those for a normal direction for the flow of blood. A ventricular septal defect is present in about 50% of the cases. S.V. = systemic ventricle; V.V. = venous ventricle.

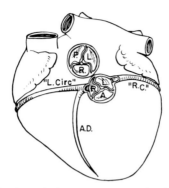

FIG. 75. Classical distribution of the coronary arteries in corrected transposition. The coronary arteries are inverted, so that the artery to the right forms the anterior descending artery (A.D.). "L. Circ" = inverted left circumflex artery; "R.C." = inverted right coronary artery.

common), the aorta is situated obliquely, ventrally, and to the left of the main pulmonary trunk. In the other type, the aorta is positioned directly ventral (anterior) to the pulmonary trunk. In both types the aortic sinuses are the anterior (noncoronary), the right, and the left (Fig. 75). The arteries arising from the right aortic sinus are an inverted left coronary artery and a second artery (inverted left circumflex) which runs in the right atrioventricular sulcus. That artery which arises from the left aortic sinus is the inverted right coronary artery. It courses in the left atrioventricular sulcus, gives rise to a marginal branch, and usually terminates as the posterior descending coronary artery.

In complete situs inversus associated with corrected transposition of the great vessels, the state is a mirror image of that in situs solitus with corrected transposition of the great vessels. With regard to the coronary arteries, the one on the left gives rise to the anterior descending and left circumflex branches, the one on the right follows the usual course of the right coronary artery in the normal heart of situs solitus.

In corrected transposition in situs solitus, the apex of the heart may lie to the right (isolated dextrocardia). This detail does not alter the origin and course of the coronary arteries from the classic patterns in corrected transposition in situs solitus.

In corrected transposition in situs inversus, the apex of the heart is expected to be on the right side. When it occurs on the left (isolated levocardia in situs inversus), the coronary arterial patterns are those classic for the basic condition, corrected transposition in situs inversus.

Right Ventricular Aorta and Biventricular Pulmonary Trunk

In this uncommon condition, the aorta arises from the right ventricle, while the pulmonary trunk arises above a ventricular septal defect from both ventricles, mainly the left.

Anatomically, this condition lies between classic complete transposition of the great vessels, on one hand, and origin of both great vessels from the right ventricle, Type II (Taussig-Bing complex), on the other. It differs from the origin of both great vessels from the right ventricle (Type II) in that in the latter condition, the pulmonary trunk which arises near a ventricular septal defect takes its origin entirely from the right ventricle; in the anomaly considered herein, the biventricular pulmonary trunk straddles a ventricular septal defect and arises mainly from the left ventricle and its valve is in continuity with the mitral valve; this feature is not present in origin of both great vessels from the right ventricle.

In both cases available to us of the condition being considered, the posteriorly positioned aortic sinus was the "noncoronary" one. In both, the main right coronary and left coronary arteries arose from the right and the left positioned aortic sinuses respectively. In one case (Fig. 76a), two anterior descending branches were present. The main one arose from the left coronary artery and ran in the anterior interventricular groove. The smaller of the two anterior descending arteries arose as a

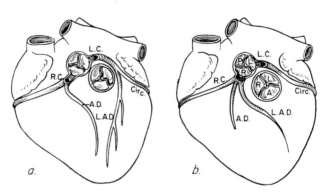

FIG. 76. Patterns of coronary arterial origin and distribution in two cases of right ventricular aorta and biventricular pulmonary trunk. *a.* There are two anterior descending coronary arteries (A.D. and L.A.D.). One originates from the right coronary and one from the left. *b.* The right coronary artery gives rise to two branches having the distribution of the anterior descending artery (A.D. and L.A.D.). The artery arising from the left aortic sinus is the left circumflex coronary artery.

branch from the right coronary artery. It crossed the outflow tract of the right ventricle to approach the anterior interventricular sulcus.

In the second case (Fig. 76*b*), two anterior descending arteries arose from the right coronary; the larger one (left anterior descending) crossed the infundibulum of the right ventricle and supplied the anterior wall of the left ventricle. The smaller one supplied the anterior wall of the right ventricle.

Common Ventricle with Transposition of the Great Vessels

As used here, the term "common ventricle" refers to the state in which there is one large receiving chamber in the heart. Anteriorly and basally, there is a subdivision of the chamber known as the "infundibulum." In common ventricle with transposition of the great vessels, the anteriorly lying transposed aorta arises from the infundibulum, while the posteriorly lying pulmonary trunk arises directly from the basal aspect of the main chamber. Whatever the atrioventricular mechanism, this leads into the main part of the common ventricle. The state of the atrioventricular valves varies. In a study of 26 cases, Elliott and associates (2) found

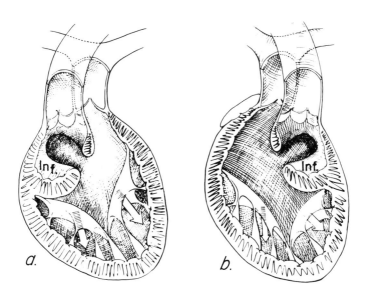

FIG. 77. Diagrammatic display of two types of common ventricle. In each, the great vessels are transposed. *a.* The infundibulum (Inf.) and aorta are noninverted. *b.* The infundibulum and aorta are inverted.

two atrioventricular valves in 11 cases, tricuspid atresia in seven, mitral atresia in five, and a common atrioventricular valve in three.

The position of the infundibulum varies and may be said to be inverted or noninverted. In the cases reported by Elliott's group from our services, these two types occurred equally often. When the infundibulum is located at the right aspect of the base of the heart, it is considered to be "noninverted." The sweep of the ascending aorta is toward the right. When the

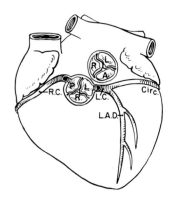

FIG. 78. Coronary arterial pattern in single ventricle without inversion of the infundibulum or transposition of the aorta. Arising from the aorta are the left and right coronary arteries, each having an essentially normal distribution. The anterior (R.) aortic sinus is the noncoronary sinus.

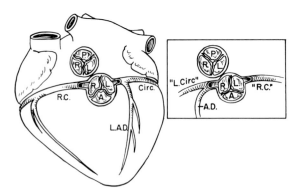

FIG. 79. Patterns of coronary arterial origin and distribution in common ventricle with inverted transposition of the great vessels. In the main body of the illustration, the coronary arteries are shown as having the usual origin and distribution. Inset: The coronary arteries are inverted as in classical transposition as shown in Fig. 75.

infundibulum is located at the left aspect of the base of the heart, it is considered "inverted" (Fig. 77). The sweep of the ascending aorta is toward the left.

The relationships between the aorta and pulmonary trunk are like those in complete transposition. In eight of our 13 cases there was an oblique relationship (Type I) and in five cases an anteroposterior pattern (Type III). The position of the aortic sinuses in all 13 cases was similar to that in complete transposition (Fig. 78). The left coronary artery arose from the left aortic sinus and branched into anterior descending and left circumflex branches. The right coronary artery arose in a right posterior position and coursed in the right atrioventricular sulcus.

With inversion of the infundibulum, the relationship of the ascending aorta and the pulmonary trunk was like that in corrected transposition. In 13 such cases that we have studied, the position of the aortic sinuses was identical to that in corrected transposition (Fig. 79). In each of these cases, the anterior aortic sinus was the noncoronary one. In nine cases, the coronary arterial pattern was identical to that seen in the normal, while in the remaining four cases, the anterior descending artery arose as a branch of the right coronary in a manner identical to that seen in corrected transposition.

Origin of Both Great Vessels from the Right Ventricle (Double-Outlet Right Ventricle)

This congenital cardiac malformation is characterized by both the aorta and the pulmonary trunk arising from the right ventricle. The only outlet for the left ventricle is a ventricular septal defect.

According to the position of the ventricular septal defect, two subdivisions were recognized by Neufeld and associates (12) (Fig. 80). In Type I the ventricular septal defect is below the crista supraventricularis; in Type II, it is above the crista (Taussig-Bing complex).

Regardless of the subdivision, in all these cases the aorta arises entirely from the right ventricle, lying to the right of the pulmonary trunk. The semilunar valves lie in the same horizontal body plane and there is no continuity between the mitral and aortic valves. The authors determined the anatomic relations between the aorta and the pulmonary trunk in 20 cases which they studied. From external view, the aorta and the pulmonary trunk occupied near-normal positions in 18 cases except that the aorta was situated slightly more anteriorly than normal and failed to curve posteriorly behind the pulmonary trunk at its base. In the other

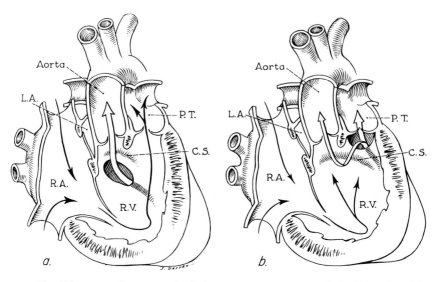

FIG. 80. Diagrammatic portrayal of the two common types of double-outlet right ventricle (origin of both great vessels from the right ventricle). *a.* Type I in which the ventricular septal defect is remote from the great vessels. *b.* Type II in which the ventricular septal defect lies in a subpulmonary position. From ref. 12.

two cases, the relation of the great vessels resembled that in the majority of cases of complete transposition as the aorta was situated to the right and more anteriorly than the pulmonary trunk.

In more than half of the cases of origin of both great vessels from the right ventricle, the coronary arterial origin and patterns were like those in normal hearts. Among the common variations from the normal, were a single coronary artery and both coronary arteries originating from one aortic sinus.

In those cases in which the origin and course of the two coronary arteries were identical to those in the normal heart, the right coronary arose from the right aortic sinus and the left coronary from the left aortic sinus. The posterior aortic sinus was the noncoronary sinus (Fig. 81*a*). In one of the cases, two anterior descending coronary arteries were present; the major one arose from the left coronary artery and the minor one from the right coronary artery.

In one case (Fig. 81*b*), a large left coronary artery arose above the left aortic sinus, and shortly after its origin it gave rise to the right coronary artery. The left coronary then continued for a short distance before

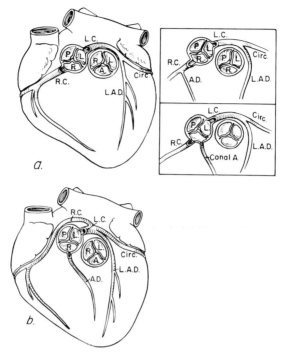

FIG. 81. Coronary arterial patterns in double-outlet right ventricle. *a.* In the main body of the illustration, an essentially normal pattern is present. Upper inset: An accessory anterior descending coronary artery (A.D.) arises from the right coronary artery. Lower inset: A large conal artery arises from the right aortic sinus anterior to the origin of the right coronary artery. *b.* Main coronary arterial system is derived from a stem originating in the left aortic sinus. From this, the right and left coronary arteries arise in turn. An accessory artery functioning as an accessory anterior descending coronary artery (A.D.) arises independently from the right aortic sinus.

branching into the left circumflex and anterior descending coronary arteries. A small accessory anterior descending artery arose independently from above the right aortic sinus and coursed down the anterior interventricular sulcus as a minor anterior descending artery.

In each of three cases, a single coronary artery was present and was associated with a bicuspid aortic valve (Fig. 82a). In one of these three cases, the single coronary artery arose from the left side of the anteriorly positioned aortic sinus and shortly after its origin gave off three main branches that followed the normal courses of the right coronary, left anterior descending and circumflex arteries, respectively.

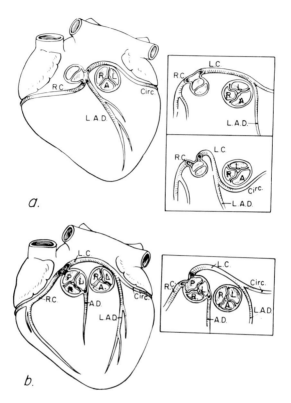

FIG. 82. Coronary arterial patterns in double-outlet right ventricle (continued).
a. Single coronary artery arising from the left side of the anterior sinus of a bicuspid
aortic valve. The vessel branches into the three standard coronary arteries. Upper
inset: A single coronary artery arising from right side of the posteriorly positioned
bicuspid aortic valve. This vessel gives rise to right and left coronary arteries.
The latter, in turn, branches into the two standard branches after coursing behind
the pulmonary trunk. Lower inset: Two coronary arteries arising from the posterior
sinus of a bicuspid aortic valve. The left coronary artery, after proceeding between
the aorta and pulmonary trunk, branches into the two standard branches; the left
circumflex artery passes anterior to the pulmonary trunk. *b.* The main coronary
arterial system arises from the posterior aortic sinus, and from this trunk, the
right and left coronary arteries arise. There is an accessory anterior descending
coronary artery (A.D.) arising from the left aortic sinus. Inset: Two separate
ostia are shown for the right and left coronary arteries in the posterior aortic
sinus, while an accessory anterior descending coronary artery arises from the left
aortic sinus.

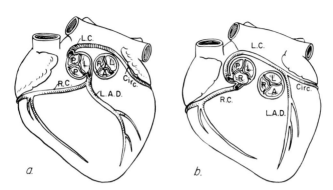

FIG. 83. Coronary arterial patterns in double-outlet right ventricle (continued). *a.* Origin of the left circumflex artery (L.C.) from the posterior aortic sinus, while the left aortic sinus gives rise to a single vessel from which the right and anterior descending coronary arteries branch. *b.* Separate ostia for the right and left coronary (L.C.) arteries from the right aortic sinus.

In each of the other two cases in which a single coronary artery was present (Fig. 82*a*), the artery originated from the right side of the posteriorly positioned aortic sinus. Shortly after its origin, it divided into the right coronary and left coronary arteries, The former proceeded to the right atrioventricular sulcus. In one of the cases, the left coronary ran behind the pulmonary trunk and in the other case between the great vessels.

In the 17th and 18th cases of double-outlet right ventricle (Fig. 82*b*), the right and left coronary arteries arose from the posterior aortic sinus (in one case from a common ostium). In each, the left coronary artery passed posterior to the pulmonary trunk before dividing into its anterior descending and left circumflex branches. In each of these cases, in addition, a relatively small anterior descending artery arose from the left aortic sinus.

In the 19th case, the left circumflex artery arose independently from the posterior aortic sinus, while a second artery arose from the left aortic sinus. The latter vessel divided into the anterior descending and right coronary arteries (Fig. 83*a*).

In the 20th case, both coronary arteries arose from the right aortic sinus. The left coronary artery proceeded around the posterior aspect of the aorta and lateral to the pulmonary trunk. In the latter location, it divided into its left circumflex and anterior descending branches (Fig. 83*b*).

Tetralogy of Fallot

In the tetralogy of Fallot, the distribution of the coronary arteries is of importance from the surgical standpoint, as variations in course of arteries may interfere with approaches to the right ventricle (8). Longenecker and associates (10) studied the coronary arteries in 22 cases of tetralogy by dissection and injection. They found that the right ventricle was more vascularized than normal but that the overall distribution was normal in 21 of 22 cases. In one case, the left coronary artery coursed between the aorta and pulmonary trunk, then passed in front of the pulmonary trunk and finally penetrated the myocardium. Among 74 surgical cases of tetralogy, Kirklin and associates (8) found one case in which only a single coronary artery was present. This was oriented as a right coronary artery. It gave off a large left branch that crossed the outflow tract of the right ventricle. In three cases, these investigators found the anterior descending artery originating from the right coronary artery, while the left circumflex artery arose independently. At operation, Senning (15) observed that among 27 patients with tetralogy, five had anomalous coronary arteries. In four of these, the anterior descending coronary artery originated from the right coronary artery and ran across the right ventricular infundibulum to reach the anterior interventricular sulcus. In the fifth case, the entire left coronary artery originated from the right coronary artery, essentially like the single coronary artery in the case reported by Kirklin and associates (8) and in another case studied at autopsy by Friedman and co-workers (5).

Gadboys and associates (6) described a case in which the anterior descending artery arose from the right coronary artery. The left circumflex artery arose independently from the aorta as a vestigial vessel.

From the laboratory of Dr. Maurice Lev, Meng and associates (11) studied 109 autopsied cases of tetralogy of Fallot and found a variety of abnormalities of the coronary arteries. These included 1) two cases of single coronary artery, 2) one case of origin of the right coronary artery from the pulmonary trunk and 3) seven cases of origin of the anterior descending from the right coronary artery. In 40% of their cases, the right conus artery was described as "remarkably long," and in nine of these, the conus artery had been divided surgically. In eight hearts, the anterior descending branch was located within the myocardium (mural artery) for most of its distal course.

Recent reports by Björk and Björk (1) and Intonti and Marchegiani

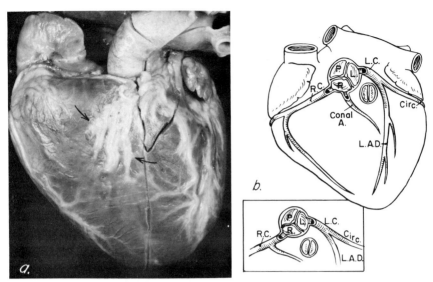

FIG. 84.   Patterns of coronary arteries in tetralogy of Fallot.   *a.* Frontal view of heart in a case of tetralogy of Fallot. A common feature is the occurrence of prominent arteries (between arrows) in the infundibular region of the right ventricle.   *b.* A prominent conal artery originating from the aorta and proceeding over the infundibulum of the right ventricle. Inset: A prominent conal artery originating from the right coronary artery.

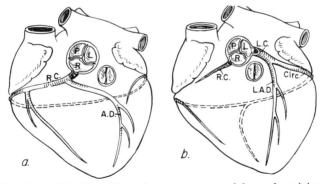

FIG. 85.   Tetralogy of Fallot with major coronary arterial supply originating from one aortic sinus.   *a.* A single coronary artery originates from the right aortic sinus and gives rise to an anterior descending branch. The right coronary artery proceeds around the base of the heart to be distributed in the territory of the left circumflex coronary artery.   *b.* The main coronary arterial supply arises from the left aortic sinus. The right coronary artery is hypoplastic and short. The major supply for the usual distribution of the right coronary artery is the left circumflex coronary artery.

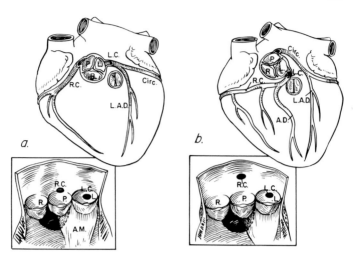

FIG. 86. Tetralogy of Fallot. Variations in origin and distribution of coronary arteries. *a.* The right and left coronary arteries arise from the posterior and left aortic sinuses, respectively. The right sinus (R.) is noncoronary. Inset: Sites of origin of coronary arteries. *b.* Independent origin of left circumflex coronary artery from the posterior aortic sinus. The vessel arising from left aortic sinus branches into anterior descending and right coronary arteries. Inset: Excessively high level of origin of the right coronary artery.

(7) have presented another variety of the coronary circulation which may be found in conjunction with tetralogy of Fallot. In these cases, a fistula formed between the left circumflex artery and the bronchial arteries. The left circumflex artery was usually dilated and tortuous.

From the available studies on tetralogy of Fallot in the literature, it appears evident that the right ventricular outflow tract is hypervascular and that major coronary arteries may cross it.

The accompanying illustrations (Fig. 84–88) portray variations in coronary arterial distribution in tetralogy of Fallot, some from our own experience and others encountered in the literature.

Robicsek and associates (13) reported a rare anomaly of the anterior descending artery. The patient, a 12-year-old girl with tetralogy of Fallot, had several variations of the coronary arteries. Only a single coronary ostium was present. This lay in the left aortic sinus. The single artery gave rise to the left circumflex branch and a vessel which crossed the right ventricular outflow tract to assume the position of the right coronary artery. No anterior descending vessel arose from either the right coronary

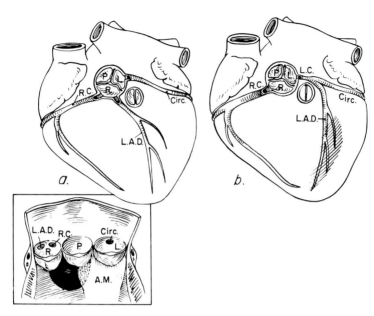

FIG. 87. Tetralogy of Fallot. Variations in patterns of origin and distribution of coronary arteries (continued). *a.* The left circumflex coronary artery arises independently from the left aortic sinus, and the right and left coronary arteries arise by independent ostia from the right aortic sinus. Inset: The relative position of the coronary ostia from the interior of the aorta. *b.* Stenosis at the origin of the left coronary artery. This was associated with scarring in the distribution of the anterior descending coronary artery.

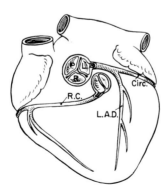

FIG. 88. Tetralogy of Fallot. Variations in patterns of origin of coronary arteries (continued). The right coronary artery arises from the pulmonary trunk, while the left coronary artery arises in the usual location from the left aortic sinus.

or the circumflex arteries; however, dissection of the anterior inter-ventricular area revealed that the anterior descending artery and vein originated from the left internal mammary artery and vein, respectively. These crossed the free pericardial space in a ligamentous band to supply the apical region of the left ventricle (Fig. 85). Two somewhat similar cases had been reported earlier by Evans (4) in 1933. In each, the anterior descending coronary artery arose from a noncardiac source, the carotid artery in one and the left subclavian artery in the other.

PERSISTENT TRUNCUS ARTERIOSUS

Van Praagh and Van Praagh (17), in 1965, reported that 28% of 57 cases (49%) of persistent truncus arteriosus studied showed coronary arterial anomalies. The anomalies were as follows: a) high ostium of the right coronary artery above the posterior sinus (11 cases); b) high ostium of

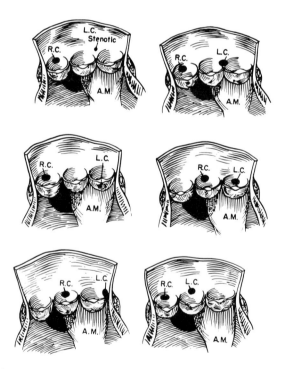

FIG. 89. Persistent truncus arteriosus. Variations in location of coronary ostia with respect to the sinuses of the truncus valve (see text). A.M. = anterior leaflet of mitral valve.

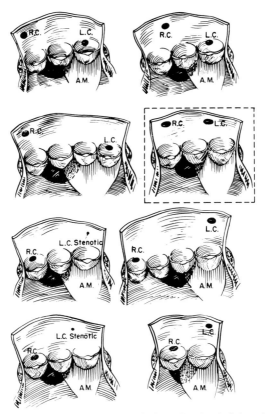

FIG. 90. Persistent truncus arteriosus. Variations in the height of origin of the coronary arteries with respect to the level of the truncus valve (see text).

the left coronary artery (five cases); c) ostium of the left coronary artery over the commissure between the left and noncoronary cusps (four cases); d) absence of right coronary artery (three cases); e) ostium of the left coronary artery above the posterior sinus (three cases); f) stenosis of the left coronary ostium (three cases); g) origin of the right coronary artery above the commissure between the right and posterior cusps (one case); h) low ostium of the left coronary artery (one case); and i) origin of the left coronary artery above the commissure between the right and left cusps (one case). Several cases exhibited more than one coronary arterial anomaly. This high incidence of variations of the coronary arteries in persistent truncus arteriosus has not been stressed in the literature.

Lampertico (9), in 1964, reviewed 49 cases of persistent truncus arte-

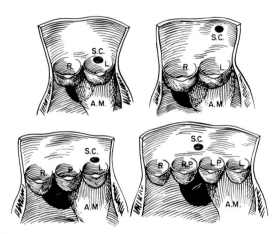

FIG. 91. Persistent truncus arteriosus. Variations in position of ostium of single coronary (S.C.) artery as seen in four cases (see text). R.P. and L.P. = right and left posterior aortic sinuses.

riosus in the files of the U.S. Armed Forces Institute of Pathology, as well as related literature. The folowing is a summary of his findings with regard to the coronary arteries (Fig. 89–91):

The right coronary artery originated from the posterior sinus in 10 instances (Fig. 89). In one of these, the left coronary arose above the commissure between the right and left cusps, and in two cases, it originated from the posterior sinus. In two other cases the ostium of the left coronary artery was above the commissure between the left and the posterior cusps; in each of these cases, however, the left coronary artery was stenotic at its origin. The ostium of the right artery was high in three cases and that of the left artery was high in five (Fig. 90). In one case both coronary ostia were high, and in another case the left coronary ostium was low.

A single (left) coronary artery was found in four of Lampertico's cases; in one the truncal valve was quadricuspid and in two, bicuspid (Fig. 91).

ANGIOCARDIOGRAPHIC EVALUATION IN TRANSPOSITION OF THE GREAT VESSELS

Angiocardiographic localization of the aortic sinuses and the origins and distribution of the coronary arteries have practical application in the diagnosis of the various types of transposition of the great vessels. We recently pointed out, however, that the angiocardiographic evaluation of the extracardiac relationship of the great vessels alone is insufficient in some cases to permit diagnosis with certainty of any particular type of transposition of the great vessels (Z. Vlodaver, V. Deutsch and H. N. Neufeld, unpublished data). Furthermore, angiographic evidence that the ascending aorta is ventral to the pulmonary trunk is not always a real diagnostic clue, since the ventrally placed aorta in respect to the pulmonary trunk may also be observed in tetralogy of Fallot or similar conditions with severe obstruction of the pulmonary flow and a dilated ascending aorta. Therefore, every additional anatomic support for the diagnosis of these various complicated conditions is of value.

We have found that evaluation of the position and relationship of the aortic sinuses and the coronary arterial pattern is helpful in the differential diagnosis in some of these cases. In addition, careful consideration of the coronary arterial pattern in transposition of the great vessels is most helpful in establishing a diagnosis. In corrected transposition of the great vessels, the anterior descending artery crosses the infundibulum of the inverted right ventricle, and this must be considered if surgical correction is undertaken. A similar situation may also be present in complete transposition of the great vessels, because the course of the left coronary artery may be in front of the left pulmonary artery rather than behind it.

Since the viewer sees the relationship of the aortic sinuses differently when the heart is *in situ* compared with that seen in the removed heart, in conformity to features seen in angiocardiographic examination the sinuses are described as viewed *in situ*. For uniformity of nomenclature, the coronary arteries, left or right, are described according to their origin and their respective anatomic ventricles.

When the great vessels are normally related, the noncoronary sinus of Valsalva is always posteriorly positioned and is usually the one that is most on the right side.

In both complete and corrected transposition of the great vessels, the sinus from which the right coronary artery arises is posteriorly positioned and the noncoronary sinus is anteriorly positioned. In complete transposition, however, the noncoronary sinus lies anteriorly and toward the right side, whereas in corrected transposition, it lies anteriorly and toward the left side. These findings are not influenced by dextroversion or levoversion.

Angiocardiographic evaluation of the origin and course of the coronary arteries has been found to be useful in the diagnosis of transposed vessels because the right coronary artery originates from the posterior aortic sinus. Furthermore, the inversion of the coronary arteries in corrected transposition has enabled us to differentiate between complete and corrected transposition.

REFERENCES

1. BJÖRK VO and BJÖRK L. Coronary artery fistula. *J Thorac Cardiovasc Surg* **49**: 921, 1965.
2. ELLIOTT LP, AMPLATZ K and EDWARDS JE. Coronary arterial patterns in transposition complexes. Anatomic and angiocardiographic studies. *Am J Cardiol* **17**: 362, 1966.
3. ELLIOTT LP, NEUFELD HN, ANDERSON RC, ADAMS P JR and EDWARDS JE. Complete transposition of the great vessels. I. An anatomic study of sixty cases. *Circulation* **27**: 1105, 1963.
4. EVANS W. Congenital stenosis (coarctation), atresia and interruption of the aortic arch: A study of 28 cases. *Q J Med* **26**: 1, 1933.
5. FRIEDMAN S, ASH R, KLEIN D and JOHNSON J. Anomalous single coronary artery complicating ventriculotomy in a child with cyanotic congenital heart disease. *Am Heart J* **59**: 140, 1960.
6. GADBOYS HL, SLONIM R and LITWAK RS. The treacherous anomalous coronary artery. *Am J Cardiol* **8**: 854, 1961.
7. INTONTI F and MARCHEGIANI C. Le fistole coronariche congenite *Ann Ital Chir* **41**: 977, 1965.
8. KIRKLIN JW, ELLIS FJ JR, MCGOON DC, DUSHANE JW and SWAN HJC. Surgical treatment for the tetralogy of Fallot by open intracardiac repair. *J Thorac Cardiovasc Surg* **37**: 33, 1959.
9. LAMPERTICO P. Persistent truncus arteriosus communis. *Folia Hered Path* (Milano) *Suppl* **4**: 1, 1964.
10. LONGENECKER CG, REEMTSMAL K and CREECH O JR. Anomalous coronary artery distribution associated with tetralogy of Fallot. A hazard in open cardiac repair. *J Thorac Cardiovasc Surg* **42**: 258, 1961.
11. MENG CC, ECKNER FA and LEV M. Coronary artery distribution in tetralogy of Fallot. *Arch Surg* **90**: 363, 1965.
12. NEUFELD HN, LUCAS RV JR, LESTER RG, ADAMS P JR, ANDERSON RC and EDWARDS JE. Origin of both great vessels from the right ventricle without pulmonary stenosis. *Br Heart J* **24**: 393, 1962.
13. ROBICSEK F, SANGER PW, DAUGHERTY HK and GALLUCCI V. Origin of the anterior interventricular (descending) coronary artery and vein from the left mammary vessels. A previously unknown anomaly of the coronary system. *J Thorac Cardiovasc Surg* **53**: 602, 1967.
14. ROWLATT UF. Coronary artery distribution in complete transposition. *JAMA* **179**: 269, 1962.
15. SENNING A. Surgical correction of transposition of the great vessels. *Surgery* **45**: 966, 1959.
16. SHAHER RM and PUDDER GC. The coronary arterial anatomy in complete transposition of the great vessels. *Am J Cardiol* **17**: 355, 1966.
17. VAN PRAAGH R and VAN PRAAGH S. The anatomy of common aortico-pulmonary trunk (truncus arteriosus communis) and its embryologic implications. A study of 57 necropsy cases. *Am J Cardiol* **16**: 406, 1965.

CHAPTER X

HISTOLOGIC PATTERNS OF THE CORONARY ARTERIES IN CHILDREN

Normal
Relation to hemodynamic stresses

The coronary arteries, unlike most organs, do not attain their maximum development at birth, but rather the intima and elastic tissue grow progressively from birth to old age.

The histologic changes which appear in the corronary arteries during the various stages of development in fetal and early extrauterine life have been studied and recognized by many authors. The question arises as to whether these early changes are pathologic or merely developmental changes in the arterial wall.

NORMAL

In fetuses, the intima of the coronary arteries is not mature, consisting of a very thin layer of endothelial cells (Fig. 92a). Immediately beneath it lies the internal elastic membrane (lamina elastica interna), which separates the intima from the media. The internal elastic membrane is always found as a prominent band of homogeneous material and is essentially a continuous tube with longitudinal corrugations. The media consists of delicate smooth muscle cells with occasional fine elastic fibrils. The adventitia is an indistinctly defined layer of collagenous connective tissue and some elastic fibers.

Postnatally, the first visible changes are seen a few days after birth and are localized in the internal elastic membrane, in the form of splitting or fragmentation. In the region of the splitting of the elastic membrane, fibroblasts proliferate. Schornagel (35) referred to these cells as stellate cells of Langhans, that is, cells of mesenchymal nature.

In the first postnatal month, splitting of the elastic membrane becomes

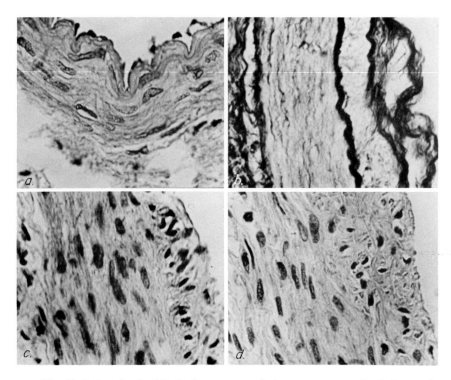

FIG. 92. Variations in the histologic structure of the coronary arteries before and after birth. *a*. From a premature stillborn female infant. A thin intima rests on the media. Hematoxylin and eosin; × 165. *b*. From an infant, two months of age. Splitting of the internal elastic membrane. Elastic tissue stain; × 235. *c*. From an infant, two months old. Fibroblastic proliferation in relation to the splitting of the internal elastic lamina shown in *b*. Hematoxylin and eosin; × 235. *d*. From an infant, one month old. The superficial part of the media shows degenerative changes of the muscle fibers. Hematoxylin and eosin; × 235.

more prominent and the adjacent smooth muscle cells of the media lose their shape and position and show degenerative changes (Fig. 92). Between the fibers of the split internal elastic membrane, smooth muscle cells begin to appear, tending to run in a longitudinal direction. In some instances, proliferation and thickening of the intimal layer are present with an increase of mucopolysaccharides under the endothelium (Fig. 93*a*).

The number of smooth muscle cells between the elements originating from the splitting of the internal elastic membrane increases and, in addition, fragmented elastic fibrils begin to appear among the ingrowing muscle

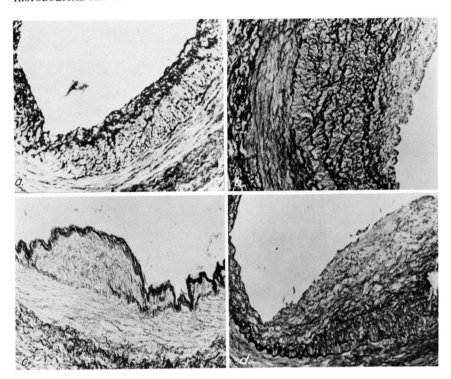

FIG. 93. Histologic structure of coronary arteries in infants. *a.* Coronary artery from a five-month-old infant stained for colloidal iron shows positive reaction at the junction of media and intima, which are sites of fibroblastic proliferation. Colloidal iron stain; × 165. *b.* Coronary artery from a six-month-old infant showing a well-developed musculo-elastic layer. Elastic tissue stain; × 235. *c.* From a three-day-old infant. Cushion-like structures in coronary artery formed by proliferated fibroelastic tissue. Elastic tissue stain; × 56. *d.* From a seven-month-old male infant. The cushion-like formation results from a well-established fibroelastic layer. Elastic tissue stain; × 56.

fibers. As a result of these changes a new layer, the musculo-elastic layer, is formed between the obvious intima and media (Fig. 93b). The new layer shows variations in distribution. In some subjects, it may have formed a complete circumferential layer at six months of age; in others of the same age, the layer may be found only in localized areas.

The intimal changes are of varying intensity, tending to increase with advancing age. In the first month, they consist of intimal cushions composed of fibroblasts and several layers of fine elastic fibers that occupy not more than half of the arterial circumference (Fig. 93c). These cushions,

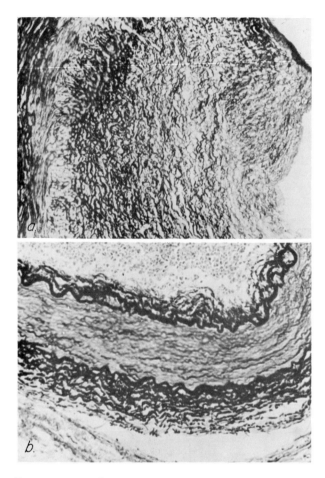

FIG. 94. *a*. Coronary artery from a seven-year-old boy showing a localized fibro-elastic layer causing asymmetrical thickening of the intima. Elastic tissue stain; × 146. *b*. From a four-month-old infant. Well-developed external elastic laminae. Elastic tissue stain; × 109.

when more diffuse, constitute the so-called fibroelastic layer in which droplets of acid mucopolysaccharides are found.

By the age of six months, the intimal thickening is more diffuse (Fig. 93*d*). At a more advanced stage, by the end of the first year, marked intimal and medial changes have led to asymmetric or diffuse thickening of the arterial wall. Beneath the intima, which is rich in collagen and elastic fibers, there is a thick musculo-elastic layer which, in some instances, may be associated with apparent loss of medial tissue leaving only two to three rows of stretched muscle cells at the periphery. At this time, the media contains more numerous connective tissue bundles and elastic fibers (Fig. 94a). In the adventitia, elastic fibers adjacent to the media show an increase in number and density and form the external elastic membrane (Fig. 94b).

From the age of six months to one year, foam cells are often present in the intima and there are small elongated spaces in the musculo-elastic layer. In sections stained with alcian blue and colloidal iron, the foam cells give a negative reaction for acid mucopolysaccharides, but the empty spaces show a positive reaction for it (39). Sudan black staining of paraffin sections also gives a negative result.

These early structural findings are essentially the same as those of other workers, beginning with Virchow (38) and continuing with Schultz (36), Wolkoff (43), Aschoff (2), Gross and associates (18), Moschcowitz (30), Moon (29), Levene (22) and Schornagel (35).

It has been believed that the most important factors affecting the normal development of the coronary arterial wall are mechanical, or metabolic, or both, in the subject as a whole and restricted to the tissues of the coronary arterial wall. Some authors have expressed the view that the dominant factor in the production of these changes is the normal intravascular pressure and that the hyperplasia of the intima and of the elastic tissue is compensatory and adaptive to the progressive increase of intraarterial pressure that normally occurs from birth to old age (2, 30).

Other investigators have stated that the earliest demonstrable change, that is, the splitting of the internal elastic membrane, represents a reaction of the vessel to an injury, that is, intravascular tension which is greater than the tensile strength of the vessel wall (29). Still others have suggested that these early lesions in the elastic membrane represent sites of underlying weakness of the media. Histologic studies, such as the counting of medial muscle fibers or the measuring of size of the nuclei, however, have not provided support for this theory (22). Other possibilities are intrauterine or extrauterine infection or anoxia but again there is no proof of the role of such factors (22, 27).

Most investigators describe the cells involved in the early structural changes as fibroblasts (2, 8, 28, 29, 42). There is a close association of fibroblastic proliferation with increase of mucoid substance (28) and the deposition of mucopolysaccharides is considered to be a manifestation of fibroblastic activity (19).

According to Haust and others (20), the cellular elements involved in the early structural alterations principally affect smooth muscle cells rather than fibroblasts. Their observations indicate that the smooth muscle cells are derived from endothelium affected by injury and that it is such cells, and not fibroblasts, which penetrate into the intima and produce the intercellular connective tissue elements. Evans (14) and Malyschew (25) have presented the same viewpoint. Stieve (37), however, postulated that the smooth muscle cells are derived from fibroblasts and Merkel (26) has suggested that the proliferating cells migrate from the media into the intima through naturally occurring gaps in the internal elastic membrane.

Smooth muscle cells which are injured experimentally may undergo alteration of both structure and function. Differentiation may occur in the direction of fibroblasts and as a result in the synthesis of collagen (31).

Another aspect of early changes that has been investigated is the role of lipid deposition in the intima of the coronary artery. A controversial point is whether or not there is a relationship between the early structural changes of the coronary wall and lipid deposition. Moon (28), Moschcowitz (30) and Dock (9) have stated that there is no such correlation, while Fangman and Hellwig (15) have stated that there is. Moon (28) found no correlation between the lipid droplets and the degree of intimal fibrosis. According to Duguid, the deposition of fibrin from the blood is responsible to some degree for the progressive intimal thickening in early life (10, 11).

Some authors have found differences in the structure of the coronary arteries between boys and girls in early life, and this early difference is believed to be one of the explanations of the predominance of coronary sclerosis in men compared with women. Some investigators have found a greater degree of intimal thickening in the male newborn (9, 15, 29), whereas others have found the sex difference only after the first month of life (22). To others, this difference is not significant (17, 24). Gross and associates (18) considered the development of the early intimal changes as a normal phenomenon and the deposition and formation in appreciable amounts of additional elements such as calcium salts, lipoid crystals, blood cells and cells of inflammation as abnormal. According to Schornagel (35) and Dock (9), the early alterations in the elastic fibers and proliferation of fibroblasts should be interpreted as a normal physiologic phenomenon of adaptation to the high demands of the coronary arteries during the first month of life. Jores (21) and Merkel (26) stated that the early changes in the internal elastic membrane are the first departure from normal and are to be considered a manifestation of arteriosclerosis and the basis for the development of the classical atheromatous lesion. Moon (29), Minkowski (27), Fangman and Hellwig (15), Gillot (17) and Pizzagalli and Bertana (33) have expressed the same opinion, namely, that early morphologic alterations after birth are early phases of the arteriosclerotic process and that it seems reasonable to consider them as manifestations of a generalized and basic tissue reaction to injury.

The later stages of hyalinization of the intima, accumulation of large amounts of lipids and calcification may well be functions of the aging process. According to Moon (29) and Lober (23), age is the most important factor in the development of coronary sclerosis. Wilens (42) suggested that the intimal thickening in early life is not a natural developmental phenomenon but is related to the formation of atherosclerotic plaques. In his opinion, the intimal changes are the result of hereditary and mechanical factors, and they provide a basis for the coronary sclerosis regularly encountered in old age. According to Moschcowitz (30), hyperplastic arteriosclerosis represents a biologic progression of the normal hyperplasia of the intima and elastica that begins at birth. Lober (23) has stated that there is no point in time at which the artery can be said to have stopped developing in growth and to have started becoming diseased. The distinction of normal and abnormal is arbitrary. Moschcowitz's criterion is visibility of the lesions; if grossly visible, the changes are abnormal.

RELATION TO HEMODYNAMIC STRESSES

The structural changes described may relate to hemodynamic stresses which occur in the coronary arteries (40) (Fig. 95).

During the first hours after birth, hydrostatic pressure in the aorta (34) increases and, parallel to this, the hydrostatic pressure in the coronary arteries rises (41). According to Laplace's law, two forces determine the equilibrium of the wall of the blood vessels. These forces are represented by the equation:

$$T = P \times r$$

where P = blood pressure; r = radius; and T = tension of the wall. Our views of the application of this law are shown diagrammatically in Fig. 96a.

Very high pressure causes instability of the equilibrium, and stretching of the vessels results. The total tension in the wall has two important components: 1) elastic tension contributed to mainly by the elastic tissue, and

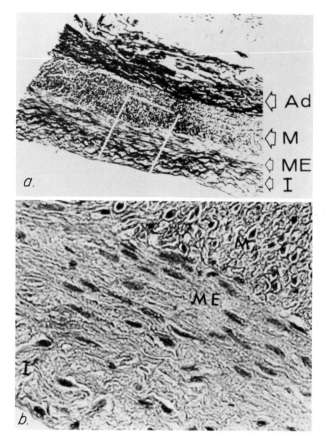

FIG. 95. *a.* Longitudinal section of a coronary artery in an infant (low-power view). The various layers are identified as follows: Ad = adventitia; M = media; ME = musculo-elastic layer; I = intima. The area within the rectangle is shown in higher power in *b.* Hematoxylin and eosin; × 73. *b.* Higher magnification of the segment of arterial wall shown in rectangle in *a.* Abbreviations correspond. Hematoxylin and eosin; × 255.

2) active tension, which depends on contraction of smooth muscle. Burton (6) has suggested a type of linkage between the smooth muscle and the fibrous and elastic network. This would confer a mechanical advantage on the vessel and would explain the ability of the vessel to withstand high blood pressure without any deformation. According to Burton (7) the pressure on the muscle cells of the musculo-elastic layer is only 1 to 2% of the actual pressure.

In view of these hemodynamic considerations, it seems that an arterial wall composed only of circular muscle cells would be unable to withstand the rise in blood pressure immediately after birth, and would therefore become deformed.

Since the musclo-elastic layer presents a network of interlacing elastic longitudinal and circular fibers (Fig. 95), we consider it an important factor in determining the total tension of the arterial wall. This layer is able to adapt to the change in blood pressure and thus avoid deformation of the arterial wall. We consider this phase to be of great importance in preserving the equilibrium of the wall and have called it the "adaptive" phase (Fig. 96b).

In more advanced stages, collagen fibers replace the fibroblasts and hyperplastic changes occur in the elastic fibers. These changes are interpreted as those of maturation, and we have referred to these collectively as the "maturity" phase. The histologic changes included in the maturity phase appear early in certain cases and are pronounced and also visible macroscopically. In the latter circumstance, the thickening may be considered as abnormal and may be called the "fibrous type of arteriosclerosis."

It is worth mentioning that the development of the musculo-elastic layer parallels the development of the intima in the epicardial coronary trunks (5, 12, 13, 16). This latter portion of the coronary artery is exposed to the aortic blood pressure during systole though coronary flow is minimal in view of the simultaneous contraction of the ventricular myocardium.

In those segments wherein the musculo-elastic layer is well developed, there is deficient development of the media. This was shown by counting the number of muscle rows. Fewer are found in the areas over prominent musculo-elastic segments.

By the visopan-planimetric method (1), it is also possible to show that over thick musculo-elastic segments the medial layer is thinner than elsewhere. This suggests that in such areas the musculo-elastic layer contributes to the integrity of the vessel wall. We were impressed by the fact that, in addition to the earliest degenerative changes (splitting) in the internal elastic membrane, changes occurred among the smooth muscle cells in these same areas. These changes took the form of disorganization of the cell, swelling of the cytoplasm, and pyknosis and karyorexis of the nuclei.

The smooth muscle cells are of primitive structure, and it is possible that they retain multipotential properties for some time after birth (3). Thus, it is possible to explain their ability to change and adapt to hemodynamic conditions which appear after birth.

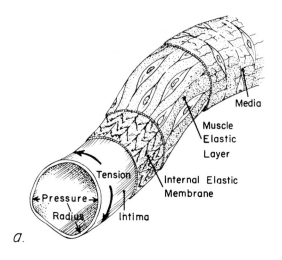

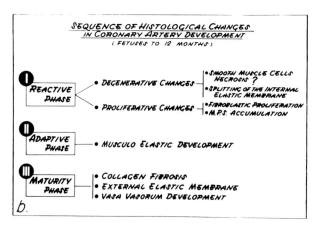

FIG. 96. *a.* Histologic structure and hemodynamic flows in the coronary artery. Note the tension in the wall of the vessel as opposed to pressure. *b.* Sequence of phases in the postnatal development of the coronary arterial structure. M.P.S. = mucopolysaccharide. From ref. 40.

Some authors have suggested that the longitudinal smooth muscle cells are derived from the endothelium (26). It seems to us that these cells originate in the connective tissue from cells at first resembling fibroblasts and that only at a later stage do they assume their final character. This idea is based on the presence of the cells not only near the internal aspect of the internal elastic membrane but also near the external aspect of the membrane where endothelial cells are lacking.

Another question which remains unanswered is whether the groups of muscle cells and elastic fibers which appear in the media are in fact longitudinal cells or whether they represent the so-called spiral muscle cells. Cells of the latter type have been well described by Bohr and associates (4) who, by using a special technique, uncoiled medial helical fibers from carotid arteries of the hog.

The Laplace law does not take into account the thickness of the vessel wall (32). This may be corrected by the following equation:

$$T = P \ (r/s)$$

where P = transmural pressure (pressure inside the vessel minus the pressure from outside the vessel); r = radius; and s = wall thickness.

Considering that the coronary arteries at birth are thin-walled cylinders with a ratio of radius-to-wall thickness of less than five, the above correction factor must be borne in mind.

REFERENCES

1. ABRAMOVICI A and NEUFELD HN. Estimation of areas of histological sections. "A visopan-planimetric method." *Isr J Med Sci* **1**: 569, 1965.
2. ASCHOFF L. "Lectures on pathology." New York, Paul B Hoeber, 1924.
3. BENNINGHOFF. Cited by Lansing AI, "The arterial wall." Baltimore, The Williams & Wilkins Co, 1959.
4. BOHR DF, GOULET PL and TAQUINI AC JR. Direct tension recording from smooth muscle of resistance vessels from various organs. *Angiology* **12**: 478, 1961.
5. BRANWOOD WA. "Modern concepts of the pathogenesis of coronary atherosclerosis." Edinburgh and London, ECS Livinstone Ltd, 1963, p 2.
6. BURTON AC. Relation of structure to function of the tissues of the wall of blood vessels. *Physiol Rev* **34**: 619, 1954.
7. BURTON AC. Properties of smooth muscle and regulation of circulation. *Physiol Rev (Suppl 5)* **42**: 1, 1962.
8. CRAWFORD T and LEVENE CI. The incorporation of fibrin in the aortic intima. *J Pathol Bacteriol* **64**: 523, 1952.
9. DOCK W. The predilection of atherosclerosis for the coronary arteries. *JAMA* **131**: 875, 1946.
10. DUGUID JB. Thrombosis as a factor in the pathogenesis of coronary atherosclerosis. *J Pathol Bacteriol* **58**: 207, 1946.
11. DUGUID JB. Thrombosis as a factor in the pathogenesis of aortic atherosclerosis. *J Pathol Bacteriol* **60**: 57, 1948.
12. EDWARDS JC, BURNSIDES C, SWARM RL and LANSING AI. Arteriosclerosis in the intramural and extramural portions of coronary arteries in the human heart. *Circulation* **13**: 235, 1956.
13. ENOS WF, HOLMES RH and BEYER JC. Pathology of coronary arteriosclerosis. *Am J Cardiol* **9**: 343, 1962.
14. EVANS G. The nature of arterio-sclerosis. *Br Med J* **1**: 454, 1927.
15. FANGMAN RJ and HELLWIG CA. Histology of coronary arteries in newborn infants. *Am J Pathol* **23**: 901, 1947.
16. GEIRINGER E. The mural coronary. *Am Heart J* **41**: 359, 1951.
17. GILLOT P. Les alterations histologiques des coronaries fetales et infantiles. *Acta Cardiol (Brux)* **17**: 145, 1962.
18. GROSS L, EPSTEIN EZ and KUGEL MA. Histology of the coronary arteries and their branches in the human heart. *Am J Pathol* **10**: 253, 1934.

19. GROSSFELD H, MEYER K and GODMAN G. Differentiation of fibroblasts in tissue culture, as determined by mucopolysaccharide production. *Proc Soc Exper Biol Med* **88**: 31, 1955.
20. HAUST MP, MORE HR and MOVAT LH. The role of smooth muscle cells in the fibrogenesis of arteriosclerosis. *Am J Pathol* **37**: 377, 1960.
21. JORES L. Wesen und Entwicklung der Arteriosklerose auf Grund anatomischer und experimenteller Untersuchungen, in: "Henke und Lubarsch: Handbuch der speziellen pathologischen Anatomie und Histologie." Berlin, Springer, v 2, 1924.
22. LEVENE CI. The early lesions of atheroma in the coronary arteries. *J Pathol Bacteriol* **72**: 79, 1956.
23. LOBER PH. Pathogenesis of coronary sclerosis. *Arch Pathol* **55**: 357, 1953.
24. LOCATELLI A and ZANCHI M. Le arterie coronaire nell'eta perinatale considerazioni sulla isto morfologia. *Folia Hered Pathol (Milano)* **6**: 11, 1957.
25. MALYSCHEW BF. Über die Reaktion des Endothels der Art. carotis des Kaninchens bei doppelter Unterbindung. *Virchows Arch [Pathol Anat]* **272**: 727, 1929.
26. MERKEL H. "Die Betheiligung der Gefässwand an der Organisation des Thrombus, mit besonderer Berücksichtigung des Endothels: Eine experimentelle Studie zugleich als Beitrag zur Endothelfrage." Habilitationsschrift. Erlangen, Junge und Sohn, 1903, p. 116.
27. MINKOWSKI WL. The coronary arteries of infants. *Am J Med Sci* **214**: 623, 1947.
28. MOON HD and RINEHART JF. Histogenesis of coronary arteriosclerosis. *Circulation* **6**: 481, 1952.
29. MOON HD. Coronary arteries in fetuses, infants, and juveniles. *Circulation* **16**: 263, 1957.
30. MOSCHCOWITZ E. Hyperplastic arteriosclerosis versus atherosclerosis. *JAMA* **143**: 861, 1950.
31. MURRAY M, SCHRODT GR and BERG HF. Role of smooth muscle cells in healing of injured arteries. *Arch Pathol* **82**: 138, 1966.
32. PETERSON LH, JENSEN RE and PARNELL J. Mechanical properties of arteries in vivo. *Circ Res* **8**: 622, 1960.
33. PIZZAGALLI GF and BERTANA V. Richerche comparative istomorfologiche sulla strutture delle coronarie nei neonati di entrambi isessi. *Osp Maggiore* **7**: 356, 1959.
34. SALING E. New findings on circulation of infant immediately after delivery. *Arch Gynaekol* **194**: 287, 1960.
35. SCHORNAGEL HE. Intimal thickening in the coronary arteries in infants. *Arch Pathol* **62**: 427, 1956.
36. SCHULTZ A. Über die Chromotropie des Gefässbindegewebes in ihrer physiologischen und pathologischen Bedeutung, insbesondere ihre Beziehungen zur Arteriosklerose. *Virchows Arch [Pathol Anat]* **239**: 415, 1922.
37. STIEVE H. Die Enge der menschlichen Gebärmuter, ihre Veränderungen während der Schwangerschaft, der Geburt und des Wochenbettes und ihre Bedeutung. *Ztschr Mikrosk Anat Forsch* **14**: 549, 1928.
38. VIRCHOW R. "Gesammelte Abhandlungen zur wissenschaftlichen Medicin." Frankfurt, AM Meidinger Sohn, 1856.
39. VLODAVER Z, ABRAMOVICI AS, NEUFELD HN and LIBAN E. Coronary arteries in Yemenites. *J Atheroscler Res* **7**: 161, 1967.
40. VLODAVER Z and NEUFELD HN. The musculo-elastic layer in the coronary arteries. A histological and hemodynamic concept. *Vasc Dis* **4**: 136, 1967.
41. WIGGERS CJ. "Physiology in health and disease," 5th edn. Philadelphia, Lea & Febiger, 1955, p 741.
42. WILENS SL. The nature of diffuse intimal thickening of arteries. *Am J Pathol* **27**: 825, 1951.
43. WOLKOFF K. Über die histologische Struktur der Coronararterien des menschlichen Herzens. *Virchows Arch [Pathol Anat]* **241**: 42, 1923.

CHAPTER XI

HISTOLOGIC FINDINGS IN EARLY LIFE IN VARIOUS ETHNIC GROUPS

Studies were performed to determine whether the differences in the prevalence of coronary atherosclerosis found among adults also may be found in early life, and, if so, whether they provide a clue to the etiology and pathogenesis of atherosclerosis. Do the early changes foreshadow later abnormality? Some steps have been taken to answer this question. Two postmortem studies, one on young German recruits during World War I and the other on young soldiers during the Korean War, showed that advanced coronary atherosclerosis was present in some of these subjects (7, 15, 17, 19). During the Korean War, Enos and associates (5) found a higher incidence of coronary atherosclerosis in American than in Chinese soldiers. Other studies have been done on younger subjects (stillborn infants, children, and young adults) to determine the basic structure of the coronary wall in various ethnic groups and its role in the subsequent development of atherosclerosis (6, 9, 16, 23, 30).

To assist in pinpointing the ethiology of atherosclerosis, the chief point of reference in many studies has been to determine whether the differences found in the degree of atherosclerotic changes in the coronary arteries were the results of ethnic or environmental factors or of the interaction of both.

Some epidemiologists have postulated that the differences in coronary atherosclerosis among population groups are related to differences in habitual nutritional patterns (10, 11, 24, 25, 26, 28). The severity of atherosclerosis has been closely associated with the proportion of total calories derived from fat and with serum cholesterol (11).

In McGill's studies (13), no conclusion was reached as to whether the type of fat or amount of cholesterol in the diet was related to the incidence of atherosclerosis. Other authors (27) have also disagreed with the theories relating fat intake to the development of arteriosclerosis, since the incidence of coronary arteriosclerosis in some ethnic groups was found to be low despite a generous intake of fat. It has been suggested that hereditary and not dietary factors might explain the low incidence of coronary arteriosclerosis in these groups (18). In addition, the apparent predisposition of some ethnic groups to aortic but not to coronary arteriosclerosis suggests the importance of factors other than dietary fats in the etiology of coronary arteriosclerosis (7).

There is no sex difference in aortic lesions in any of the geographic groups studied. The aorta seems to respond differently to the etiologic

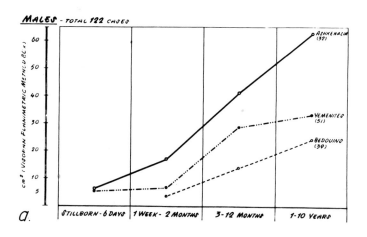

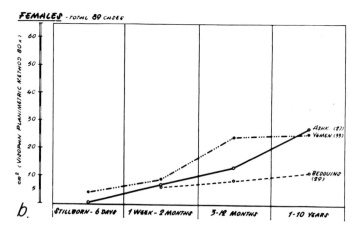

FIG. 97. Variations in thickness of intima and musculo-elastic layer of coronary arteries in three ethnic groups as follows: Ashkenazy Jews, Yemenite Jews, and Bedouins. Mean values at varying ages. a. In males. b. In females. From ref. 30.

agents of atherosclerosis than do the coronary arteries (28). One of the most important factors influencing coronary arteriosclerosis is sex. The reason is not clear.

The predominance of intimal development seen in early life in the male as contrasted to the female in the Ashkenazy group in Israel by Neufeld and Vlodaver (16) is similar to that found among American children by Dock (2) and among European children by Schornagel (22) and is consistent with the well-known sex differences in the severity of coronary arteriosclerosis. In the populations of Oslo, Norway (13), and New Orleans, United States, advanced atherosclerotic lesions were found to be more extensive in the young male than in the young female. The lack of sex differences in the intimal development in the Yemenite and Bedouin groups in Israel is similar to that in other ethnic groups such as Nigerian children. In each of these three population groups, incidence of coronary heart disease is low (20, 30).

Differences in the quantity and intensity of the intimal changes between the sexes and among various ethnic groups are found even in early life (16). These differences are apparent soon after birth but are more obvious at the end of the first year of life.

Vlodaver and co-workers (30) performed histologic examination on 211 consecutive hearts from fetuses and children up to 10 years of age in three different ethnic groups residing in Israel, namely, Ashkenazy Jews, Yemenite Jews, and Bedouins. The ratio of the cross-sectional area of the intima plus that of the musculo-elastic layer to the total cross-sectional

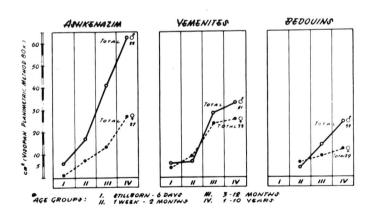

FIG. 98. Comparison of thickness of intima and musculo-elastic layer in coronary arteries in males and females of three ethnic groups. From ref. 30.

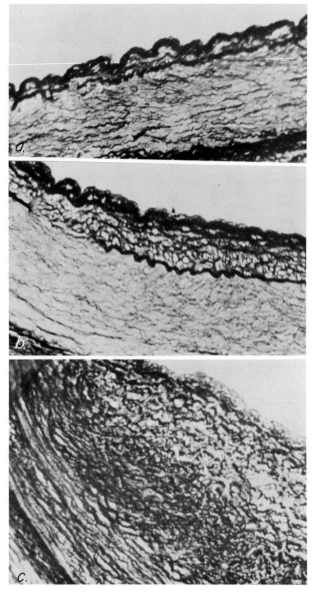

FIG. 99. Representative picture of variations of intima and musculo-elastic layer of coronary artery. *a.* From a female Bedouin, two years of age. The fibroelastic layer is thin. Elastic tissue stain; × 74. *b.* From a nine-year-old male Yemenite Jew. The intimal layer is distinct and has moderate thickening. Elastic tissue stain; × 74. *c.* From a seven-year-old Ashkenazy male subject. Major thickening of intimal layer. Elastic tissue stain; × 74.

area of the vessel was calculated. For each individual three arteries were measured. The Ashkenazy males were found to have more intima and musculo-elastic tissue than the Bedouin or Yemenite males (Fig. 97a). Such differences were not present among the females (Fig. 97b). Ashkenazy males also clearly had more intima and musculo-elastic tissue than females of this group (Fig. 98). No differences were found between the right and left coronary arteries in any of the ethnic groups.

Changes in the internal elastic membrane and the elastic fibers of the intima were less apparent in the Bedouin group than in the Ashkenazy and Yemenite Jews. In the Bedouins, in the one- to 10-year age group and particularly in the females, an intact internal elastic membrane was a common finding, and elastic fiber changes in the intima were moderate (Fig. 99a). In the Bedouins, it appears that the initial elastic changes do not become more pronounced with age, as they do in the other ethnic groups. The intima of the Ashkenazy males develops in an eccentric form and has a richer collagenous tissue component than that of the children in the Yemenite and Bedouin groups (Fig. 99b and c).

These differences in the findings between sexes and ethnic groups in children up to 10 years of age are consistent with the known differences in the prevalence of coronary arteriosclerosis and atherosclerosis, coronary heart disease and myocardial infarction in the corresponding adult populations. There is a significant difference in prevalence and severity of arteriosclerosis in the Ashkenazy group compared with the non-Ashkenazy ethnic groups studied beyond the age of 50 years (29) which correlates with alterations seen in the young.

A long-term epidemiologic study of ischemic heart disease in Israel, and an analysis of the adjusted rates for the diagnostic categories of angina pectoris and history of heart attack by location of birth shows that the Central and East European (Ashkenazy) Jews have the highest rate of the disease. Jews born in the Middle East, including Yemen and North Africa, have the lowest rates, whereas the Jews born in Southeast Europe and Israel form an intermediate group (14).

Other studies made in Israel (3, 4, 20, 21) indicate higher rates of myocardial infarction in males from Europe (Ashkenazy origin) compared with those from Asia and Africa. Higher rates in males than in females have also been found in the European-born but not in those born in Asia. Myocardial infarction is particularly rare among the Bedouins (8).

Groom and associates (9) compared the degree of intimal thickening of the coronary arteries in black Haitian and black American subjects of both sexes up to the age of 10 years; the findings were given as the average percentage of encroachment of the lumen. The results showed that the black Americans (1) have more developed and thickened intima than do the black Haitians. The dissimilarities observed in the coronary vessels of black children were predominantly variations in the degree of progression of the basic process. These differences between children of the same ethnic groups living in these two countries parallel the differences in the incidence of coronary atherosclerosis and coronary heart disease found in the corresponding adult groups (9).

According to Lansing's theory (12), changes in the elastic tissue of the intima precede the development of atherosclerosis. The low incidence of coronary atherosclerosis in adult Bedouins may, therefore, be related to the absence of elastic changes in infancy. Studies based on elastic tissue staining and micro-incineration techniques show that the elastic elements of the coronary arteries in black subjects manifest less tendency to fragment than do the corresponding elements in white subjects. This finding is consistent with the lower prevalence of coronary heart disease in black people.

It seems appropriate to assume that an intrinsic factor, probably inherited, determines the stages for maturation of the cellular and collagenous components of the intima. This would explain sex differences in the formation of collagen tissue seen in the coronary arteries of male and female children in the Ashkenazy (30), European (22) and American (2) groups.

REFERENCES

1. BLACHE JO and HANDLER FP. Coronary artery disease. A comparison of the rates and patterns of development of coronary arteriosclerosis in the Negro and white races with its relation to clinical coronary artery disease. *Arch Pathol* **50**: 189, 1950.
2. DOCK W. The predilection of atherosclerosis for the coronary arteries. *JAMA* **131**: 875, 1946.
3. DREYFUSS F. The incidence of myocardial infarctions in various communities in Israel. *Am Heart J* **45**: 749, 1953.
4. DREYFUSS F, HAMOSH P, ADAM YG and KALLNER B. Coronary heart disease and hypertension among Jews immigrated to Israel from the Atlas mountain region of North Africa. *Am Heart J* **62**: 470, 1961.
5. ENOS WF, HOLMES RH and BEYER JC. Pathology of coronary arteriosclerosis. *Am J Cardiol* **9**: 343, 1962.
6. FLORENTIN RA, LEE KT, DAOUD AS, DAVIES JN, HALL EW and GOODALE F. Geographic pathology of arteriosclerosis: A study of the age of onset of significant coronary arteriosclerosis in adult Africans and New Yorkers. *Exp Mol Pathol* **2**: 103, 1963.
7. FRENCH AJ and DOCK W. Fatal coronary arteriosclerosis in young soldiers. *JAMA* **124**: 1233, 1944.

8. GROEN JJ, BALOGH M, LEVY M and YARON E. Nutrition of the Bedouins in the Negev Desert. *Am J Clin Nutr* **14**: 37, 1964.

9. GROOM D, MCKEE EE, ADKINS W, PEAN V and HUDICOURT E. Developmental patterns of coronary and aortic atherosclerosis in young Negroes of Haiti and the United States. *Ann Intern Med* **61**: 900, 1964.

10. KEYS A, KIMURA N, KUSUKAWA A, BRONTE-STEWART B, LARSEN N and KEYS MH. Lessons from serum cholesterol studies in Japan and Los Angeles. *Ann Intern Med* **48**: 83, 1958.

11. KEYS A, BRONTE-STEWART B, BROCK JF, MOODIE A, KEYS MH and ANTONIS A. Atherosclerosis, serum cholesterol and beta lipoproteins and the diet in three populations in Cape Town. *Circulation* **12**: 492, 1955.

12. LANSING AI. The role of elastic tissue in the formation of the arteriosclerotic lesion. *Ann Intern Med* **36**: 39, 1952.

13. MCGILL HC. "The geographic pathology of atherosclerosis." Baltimore, Williams and Wilkins Co, 1968.

14. MEDALIE JH and NEUFELD HN. The Israel ischemic heart disease project. *Proc Tel-Hashomer Hosp* **3**: 41, 1967.

15. MÖNCKEBERG JG. Über die Atherosklerose der Kombattanten nach Obduktionbefunden. *Zbl Herz Gefässkr* **7**: 7, 1915.

16. NEUFELD HN and VLODAVER Z. Structural changes in the coronary arteries of infants. *Bull Ass Cardiol Ped Europ* **4**: 35, 1968.

17. NEWMAN M. Coronary occlusion in young adults; review of 50 cases in the services. *Lancet* **ii**: 409, 1946.

18. PAGE IH, LEWIS LA and GILBERT J. Plasma lipids and proteins and their relationship to coronary disease among Navajo Indians. *Circulation* **13**: 675, 1956.

19. POE WD. Fatal coronary artery disease in young men. *Am Heart J* **33**: 76, 1947.

20. ROBERTSON JH. The significance of intimal thickening in the arteries of the newborn. *Arch Dis Child* **35**: 588, 1960.

21. SAKS MI and VLODAVER Z. An autopsy study of myocardial infarction in Israel. *Pathol Microbiol* **30**: 570, 1967.

22. SCHORNAGEL HE. Intimal thickening in the coronary arteries in infants. *Arch Pathol* **62**: 427, 1956.

23. SCOTT RF, FLORENTIN RA, DAOUD AS, MORRISON ES, JONES RM and HUTT NSR. Coronary arteries of children and young adults: A comparison of lipids and anatomic features in New Yorkers and East Africans. *Exp Mol Pathol* **5**: 12, 1966.

24. SNAPPER I. Nutrition and nutritional diseases in the Orient. *Adv Intern Med* **2**: 577, 1947.

25. STAMLER J. "Lectures on preventive cardiology." New York, Grune & Stratton, 1967.

26. STEINER PE. Necropsies on Okinawans: Anatomic and pathologic observations. *Arch Pathol* **42**: 359, 1946.

27. STOUT C, MORROW J, BRANDT EN JR and WOLF S. Unusually low incidence of death from myocardial infarction. *JAMA* **188**: 845, 1964.

28. TOOR M, KATCHALSKY A, AGMON J and ALLALOUF P. Serum lipids and atherosclerosis among Yemenite immigrants in Israel. *Lancet* **i**: 1270, 1957.

29. UNGAR H and LAUFER A. Necropsy survey of atherosclerosis in the Jewish population of Israel. *Pathol Microbiol (Basel)* **24**: 711, 1961.

30. VLODAVER Z, KAHN HA and NEUFELD HN. The coronary arteries in early life in three different ethnic groups. *Circulation* **39**: 541, 1969.

CHAPTER XII

HISTOLOGIC FINDINGS IN CORONARY ARTERIES IN CONGENITAL HEART DISEASE AND METABOLIC DISEASE

Changes related to congenital heart disease
  Supravalvular aortic stenosis
  Coarctation of the aorta
  Pulmonary atresia and intact ventricular septum
  Aortic atresia and intact ventricular septum
Changes related to metabolic disease
  Gargoylism (Hurler's syndrome)
  Xanthomatosis
  Homocystinuria
  Progressive muscular dystrophy
  Calcification of the coronary arteries
  Progeria (dwarfism)
  Cystic medial necrosis

Congenital conditions may yield histologic alterations in the coronary arteries. Some of these conditions are types of congenital heart disease while others are systemic metabolic disease.

CHANGES RELATED TO CONGENITAL HEART DISEASE

Two types of congenital heart disease may be represented: 1) those primarily of anomalous origin or communication of the coronary arteries and 2) those primarily in the heart, other than the coronary arteries.

The primary changes occur in the coronary arteries proximal to anomalous communications with a cardiac chamber or in the normally arising coronary artery when the other artery arises from the pulmonary trunk (15). These changes consist of marked thickening of the media with prominent muscle bundles interspersed with numerous elastic fibers. Nonspecific local fibrous intimal thickening may also be present (Fig. 100).

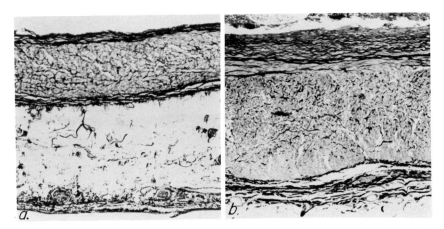

FIG. 100. Variations in structure of coronary arteries in anomalous origin of left coronary artery from pulmonary trunk. *a.* Anterior descending coronary artery. The media is thin. Elastic tissue stain; × 55. *b.* The right coronary artery. The media is thicker than in *a* and the intima shows nonspecific fibroelastic thickening. Elastic tissue stain; × 55.

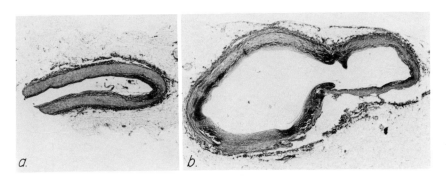

FIG. 101. Hypoplasia of coronary arteries. Origin of each coronary artery from the aorta. *a.* The right coronary artery is relatively thin-walled and shows a narrow lumen. Elastic tissue stain; × 9. *b.* The left main coronary artery. The diameter is greater than in *a* and there is nonspecific minimal fibrous thickening of the intima. Elastic tissue stain; × 9.

A second type of primary change is found in hypoplasia of one of the coronary arteries; its wall is relatively thin and the lumen is narrow (Fig. 101).

Secondary changes in the coronary arteries may occur in the presence of certain congenital anomalies primarily in the heart when hypertension is present in the coronary arteries. These consist of nonspecific intimal changes in the coronary arteries of children and atherosclerosis in young adults (16, 25). The media of the coronary arteries is thickened and elastic changes are evident. These secondary changes are particularly well developed in supravalvular aortic stenosis of the ascending aorta.

Supravalvular Aortic Stenosis

In 1962, Neufeld and associates (16) reported the necropsy findings in a two-year-old boy with uniform narrowing of the ascending aorta, a condition that may be termed the "hypoplastic type" of supravalvular aortic stenosis. In the coronary arteries, the media was thickened and contained coarse elastic fibers. These changes were attributed to systolic hypertension in the coronary vessels (Fig. 102).

In the hourglass type of supravalvular aortic stenosis, the lesion may involve the coronary ostia, and in rare cases, the free edge of an aortic cusp may be adherent to the thickened aortic intima (Fig. 103). The process results in exteriorization of the lumen of the involved coronary artery from the aortic lumen.

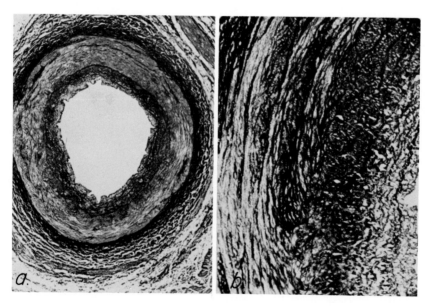

FIG. 102. Coronary arterial changes in the hypoplastic type of supravalvular aortic stenosis. There is medial hypertrophy along with splitting of the internal elastic membrane. *a.* Elastic tissue stain; × 40. *b.* Elastic tissue stain; × 100. From ref. 15.

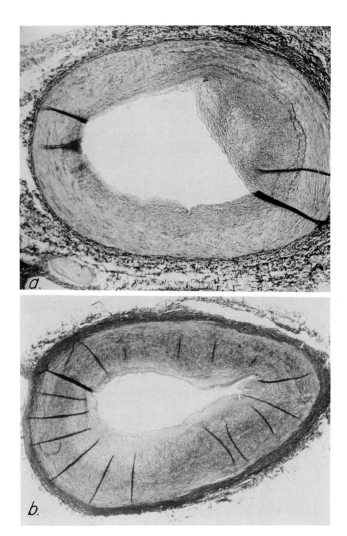

FIG. 103. Coronary arteries in hourglass type of supravalvular aortic stenosis. *a.* From a 38-year-old woman. Thickening of the media and a well-developed musculo-elastic layer and an atheromatous lesion. Elastic tissue stain; × 15. *b.* From a seven-year-old boy. Hypertrophy of the media is a prominent feature. Elastic tissue stain; × 15.

Another effect of localized supravalvular aortic stenosis is that the aortic lesion may secondarily obstruct the coronary artery at its origin (Fig. 104). A specimen of this type was shown to us by Dr. A. E. Baker. It was from a 15-month-old girl who had had a myocardial infarc-

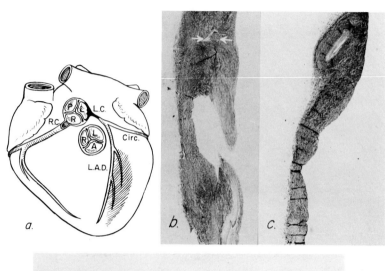

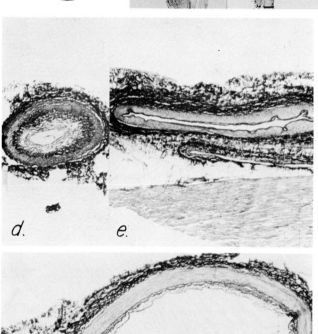

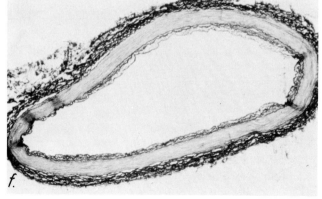

tion suggesting anomalous origin of the left coronary artery from the pulmonary trunk. Necropsy showed that both coronary arteries arose from the aorta, but on histologic examination, occlusion of the main left coronary artery was present while its two branches were patent.

The lumen of the aorta was not obstructed, but a shallow protrusion was related to the occluded left coronary ostium. Histologically, the aortic media showed a mosaic pattern like that seen in classic examples of supravalvular aortic stenosis.

Coarctation of the Aorta

Changes in the coronary arteries in 15 cases of coarctation of the aorta have been correlated with the hemodynamics of this malformation (Fig. 105). Marked intimal changes are present in the form of degenerative and proliferative changes of the elastic fibers and an excess of collagenous tissue (Fig. 106a). The media was remarkably thickened with rich elastic fibers interspersed between the muscle bundles (Fig. 106b to 108a). The media was more prominent than normal (Fig. 107). Thickening of the media was also present in the intramural coronary arteries and in the small epicardial branches (Fig. 108b). In young men with coarctation, atherosclerotic lesions of the coronary arteries were also conspicuous (Fig. 109). These coronary changes were different from those observed in young adolescents with systemic acquired hypertension.

With long-standing nephrosis and hypertension, the coronary arteries show extensive atheromatous sclerosis like that in adults. These changes are associated with medial disorganization. In coarctation of the aorta, the coronary capacity is larger than normal; this has been confirmed by the

---

FIG. 104. Severe obstruction of left coronary artery in a case of *forme fruste* supravalvular aortic stenosis. *a.* Diagrammatic portrayal of the location and extent of the lesions. *b.* The left coronary artery (between arrows) as it proceeds through the aortic wall is virtually obliterated. The aortic media shows a mosaic pattern. Elastic tissue stain; × 9. *c.* Longitudinal section. The left coronary artery has emerged from the aorta and the lumen is narrow. Elastic tissue stain; × 9. *d.* The left coronary artery after emerging from the aortic wall shows a hypoplastic character and a lumen narrowed by intimal fibrous proliferation. Elastic tissue stain; × 29. *e.* The anterior descending coronary artery. The vessel is hypoplastic but otherwise its structure is normal. Hematoxylin and eosin; × 29. *f.* The right coronary artery. The lumen is considerably wider than that of the left coronary system. Elastic tissue stain; × 26.

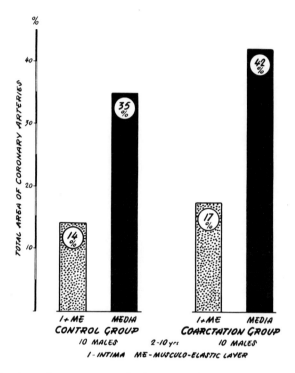

FIG. 105. Structure of coronary arteries in coarctation of aorta. Relation of intima, media, and musculo-elastic layer to the total area of coronary arteries. From ref. 25.

measurements of the external diameter (25). The total area of the vessel and of its lumen is greater than in controls (Fig. 110).

Pulmonary Atresia and Intact Ventricular Septum (Fig. 111a to c)

In 1951, Williams and associates (28) reported the finding of an anomalous vessel arising from the right ventricle in a case of pulmonary atresia with intact ventricular septum. This anomalous vessels communicated, on one hand, with the right ventricular chamber by means of myocardial sinusoids and, on the other hand, with a normal coronary arterial and capillary tree. Williams' group suggested that the anomalous coronary vessel was derived from embryonal sinusoids. In their case, injection of water and an aqueous suspension of dye into the unopened right ventricular chamber was followed by ballooning of the anomalous vessel and then by filling of the coronary arterial branches.

In 12 cases of pulmonary atresia and intact ventricular septum reported

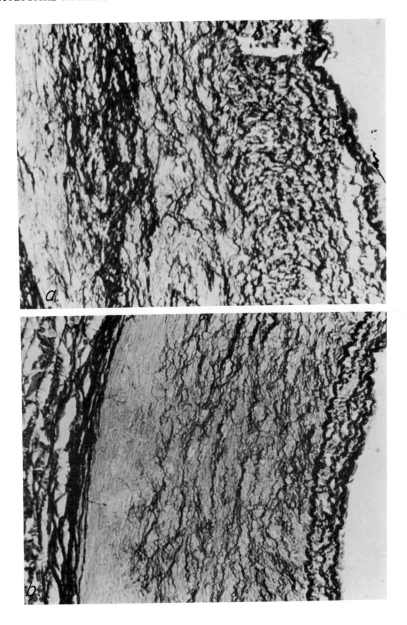

FIG. 106.   Histologic structure of coronary arteries in coarctation of aorta.   *a*. From a five-year-old boy. Marked intimal thickening with collagen and elastic tissue. Elastic tissue stain, × 90.   *b*. From a two-year-old boy. Medial thickening. Elastic tissue stain; × 90.

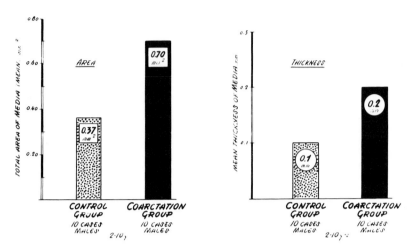

FIG. 107. Structure of coronary arteries in coarctation of aorta. Mean values for medial area and thickness. From ref. 25.

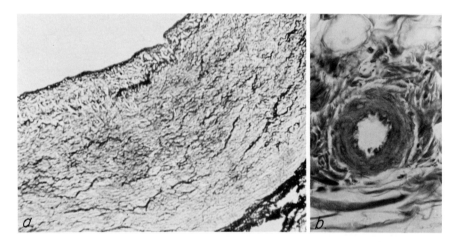

FIG. 108. Structure of coronary arteries in coarctation of the aorta. *a.* Elastosis of the media. Elastic tissue stain; × 150. *b.* Medial thickening of a small intra-myocardial artery. Hematoxylin and eosin; × 225.

by Elliott and associates (5) in 1963, a gross communication between a coronary artery and the right ventricle was present in four cases. In those cases, the tricuspid valve was functionally competent.

In each case, the right ventricular chamber was small. Enlarged sinusoids

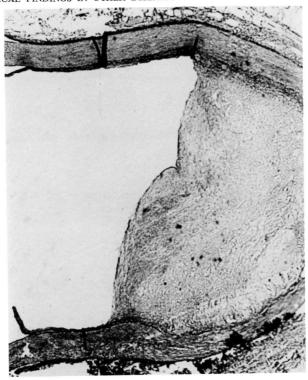

FIG. 109. Coronary arterial changes in coarctation of the aorta. Left coronary artery from a 30-year-old Yemenite Jew. Prominent atherosclerotic plaque narrows the lumen.

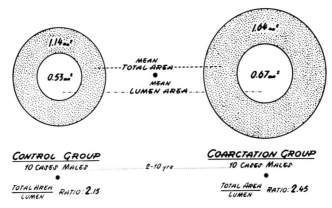

FIG. 110. Structure of coronary arteries in coarctation of the aorta. Mean total areas of media and lumen. From ref. 25.

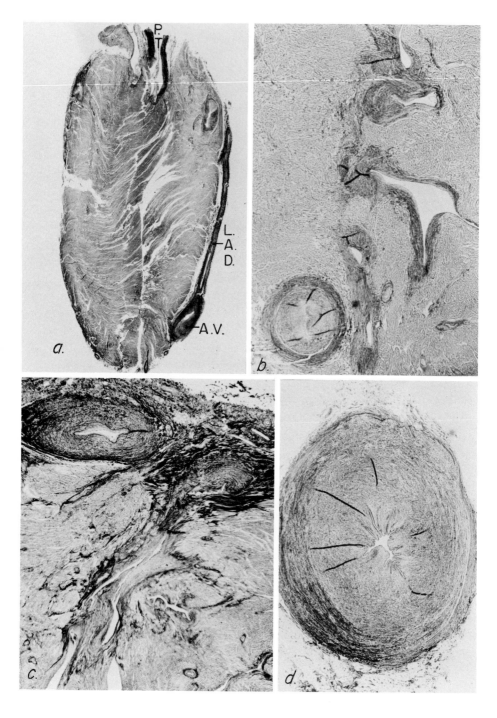

penetrated the right ventricular myocardium and converged near the epicardium where they continued as a single vessel. This anomalous vessel communicated with the left anterior descending artery at the inferior aspect of the heart, where a "dimple" was present. The coronary artery that participated in the communication was dilated and tortuous.

In classic cases of pulmonary atresia with intact ventricular septum, ostia of enlarged sinusoids are seen in the right ventricular endocardium. The myocardial sinusoids, which open into the right ventricular cavity, pass through the myocardium to reach smaller sinusoidal structures. The sinusoidal wall is thin and composed of collagen and elastic fibers covered

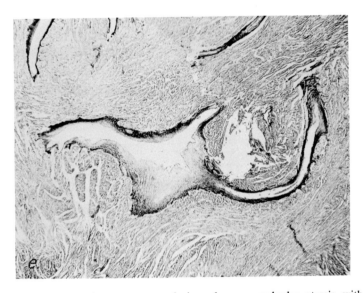

FIG. 111. Structure of coronary vessels in pulmonary valvular atresia with intact ventricular septum. a. Longitudinal section through the ventricular septum showing the anterior descending coronary artery (L.A.D.) and the origin of the pulmonary trunk (P.T.) A large anomalous vessel (A.V.) is cut in cross section. This lies near the anterior descending coronary artery but communications with the latter were not identified. Elastic tissue stain; × 2. b. Intramyocardial sinusoids are enlarged and show intimal thickening. Elastic tissue stain; × 19. c. Within the epicardium, large anomalous vessels have walls that are composed of laminations of collagen and elastic tissue and appear to be connected with intramyocardial sinusoids. Elastic tissue stain; × 19. d. Within the epicardium, an anomalous vessel has a wall composed of elastic tissue and collagen. This vessel appears to have communicated with intramyocardial sinusoids. Elastic tissue stain; × 16. e. Myocardium. Numerous dilated sinusoids showing intimal proliferation. Elastic tissue stain; × 16.

by endothelium. Minimal-to-moderate subendothelial fibrous proliferation is common in the myocardial sinuosids (Fig. 111*b*). Communication of the myocardial sinusoids with an anomalous vessel could be demonstrated in six of the nine cases with pulmonary atresia which we have had the opportunity to study by consecutive histologic sections (26) (Fig. 111*c*).

The anomalous vessels which received sinusoids are circular in cross section. The thick wall is composed essentially of collagenous fibers and numerous circular elastic fibers (Fig. 111*d* and *e*). No smooth muscle cells could be identified. The adventitia is very thick and rich in elastic fibers. Such an anomaly was identified in each of our nine cases with pulmonary atresia and small right ventricle. In seven of the nine cases, subendothelial fibrous proliferation caused near occlusion of the anomalous vessels. In most of the cases we identified anomalous vessels running near branches of the coronary arteries. A communication of an anomalous vessel with coronary arteries was demonstrated by histologic section in four cases. The coronary arteries were of normal size and, in a few cases. mild intimal fibrous thickening was seen.

The basis for enlarged myocardial sinusoids needs consideration. In pulmonary atresia, intact ventricular septum and competent tricuspid valve with right ventricular hypertension are present. Because of the elevated pressure within the right ventricular cavity, sinusoids normally present are used to carry blood out of the right ventricular cavity. Their enlargement is explained upon the basis of use. The severe intimal changes of the anomalous vessel may represent a reactive process of the vessel to the high systolic pressure under these circumstances. Whether these anomalous vessels are original sinusoids or represent persistence of fetal functional vessels remains a question.

Aortic Atresia and Intact Ventricular Septum (*Fig. 112*)

The hemodynamics of the left ventricle in aortic atresia appear to be similar to those of the right ventricle in pulmonary atresia. Grossly, in aortic atresia, one may identify enlarged ostia of sinusoids in the left ventricular endocardium. While enlarged sinusoids are readily identified in the left ventricular wall, we could not find a large anomalous vessel among the five cases studied. Characteristically, in aortic atresia the epicardial coronary arterial trunks are enlarged and tortuous; this finding suggests excess flow in these vessels (Fig. 112*a*). While the source of the excess flow may be the left ventricle, we have not yet been able to demonstrate such a pathway (Fig. 112*b*).

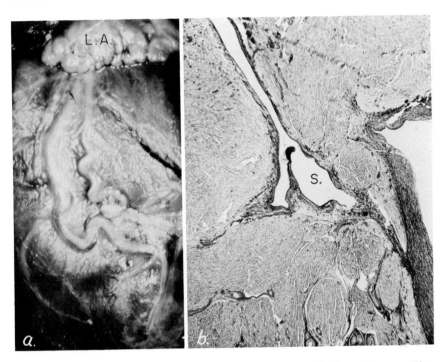

FIG. 112. Coronary vessels in aortic atresia with intact ventricular septum. *a.* The exterior of the left ventricle showing enlarged and tortuous coronary arteries. L.A. = left atrial appendage. *b.* Photomicrograph of left ventricle. Beneath the endocardium, thickened with elastic tissue, is an enlarged myocardial sinusoid (S.). Elastic tissue stain; × 17.5.

In a rare case of aortic atresia, Raghib and associates (17) demonstrated an arteriovenous fistula between the left circumflex coronary artery and the coronary sinus. The case suggested that sinusoids carried blood from the left ventricle to the left circumflex artery, whence by way of the fistula blood was directed into the right atrium.

CHANGES RELATED TO METABOLIC DISEASE
Gargoylism (Hurler's Syndrome)

In this condition the coronary arteries may be affected by deposition of macromolecular lipoprotein in the intima. The intimal layer is thickened with swollen fibroblasts, dense collagen fibers, and increased interstitial material. Coronary insufficiency may result (11, 20) (Fig. 113).

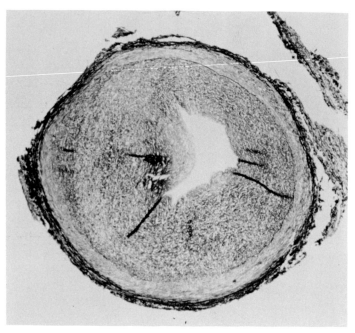

FIG. 113. Photomicrograph of coronary artery in Hurler's syndrome. Major thickening of intima. Elastic tissue stain; × 20.

Xanthomatosis

Abnormal deposition of lipids in the intima of the coronary arteries in xanthomatosis is accompanied by an abnormally high concentration of lipids in the blood. The lipid accumulation may consist of cholesterol in cases of hypercholesterolemia or of neutral fat in cases of hyperlipemia (8). Angina pectoris is frequent in these cases and was noted in young children (14, 18, 27).

Homocystinuria

In cases of this type the coronary arteries reveal intimal thickening and increased ground substance in the media with secondary changes in the smooth muscle cells (2, 19).

Progressive Muscular Dystrophy

Small coronary arteries in these cases may reveal intimal fibrous thickening and the media may show degenerative changes (7).

Calcification of the Coronary Arteries

The process essentially consists of idiopathic medial necrosis with subsequent calcification of the coronary arteries. Many etiologic factors are mentioned: hypoxia, allergic reaction, and abnormal calcium metabolism (1, 3, 10, 13, 22, 23, 24). It occurs in families, is frequently associated with endocardial fibroelastosis, and commonly involves the pulmonary arteries, renal arteries and large arteries of the extremities as well. The media of the coronary arteries shows necrotic smooth muscle cells and elastic fibers, and the lumen of the vessel is occluded by intimal proliferation (10, 13, 22).

Progeria (dwarfism)

In the rare syndrome of congenital dwarfism (progeria), the usual cause

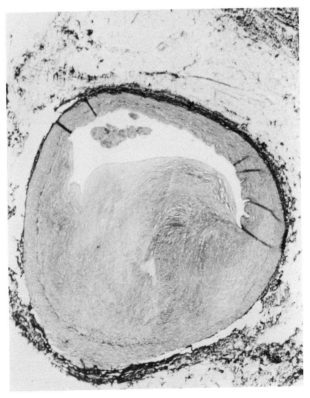

FIG. 114. Photomicrograph of coronary artery in Marfan's syndrome. Major thickening of intima with connective tissue containing a mucoid matrix. Elastic tissue stain; × 16.

of death in very early life is generalized arteriosclerosis. In those who survive to late childhood and adolescence, cardiac complications such as myocardial infarction, are common (4, 6, 9, 12, 21).

Cystic Medial Necrosis

In our experience, cystic medial necrosis of the aorta as seen in arachnodactyly (Marfan's syndrome) may be associated with coronary arterial thickening. A most extreme example was observed in a 14-year-old boy who died of dissecting aneurysm of the aorta. The coronary arteries showed severe focal intimal thickening with fibrous tissue in which stainable fat was present and was associated with change of cystic nature in the media (Fig. 114). In other cases of cystic medial necrosis of the aorta, we have observed qualitatively similar lesions, but none with the severity of this particular case.

REFERENCES

1. BRYANT JH and WHITE WH. A case of calcification of the arteries and obliterative endarteritis, associated with hydronephrosis, in a child aged six months. *Guys Hosp Rep* s. 3, **40**: 17, 1901.
2. CARSON NAJ, DENT CE, FIELD CMB and GAULL GE. Homocystinuria: clinical and pathological review of ten cases. *J Pediatr* **66**: 565, 1965.
3. CHOFFAT J-M. Morphogénèse de la médiocalcinose artérielle du nourrisson. *Cardiologia* **49**: 277, 1966.
4. COOKE JV. The rate of growth in progeria; with report of 2 cases. *J Pediatr* **42**: 26, 1953.
5. ELLIOTT LP, ADAMS P JR and EDWARDS JE. Pulmonary atresia with intact ventricular septum. *Br Heart J* **25**: 489, 1963.
6. GILFORD H. Infantilism and senilism. *Br Med J* **2**: 1408, 1902.
7. JAMES TN. An etiologic concept concerning the obscure myocardiopathies. *Progr Cardiovasc Dis* **7**: 43, 1964.
8. JENSEN J, BLANKENHORN DH and KORNERUP V. Coronary disease in familial hypercholesterolemia. *Circulation* **36**: 77, 1967.
9. KEAY AJ, OLIVER MF and BOYD GS. Progeria and atherosclerosis. *Arch Dis Child* **30**: 410, 1955.
10. LEV M, CRAENEN J and LAMBERT EC. Infantile coronary sclerosis with atrioventricular block. *J Pediatr* **70**: 87, 1967.
11. LINDSAY S. The cardiovascular system in gargoylism. *Br Heart J* **12**: 17, 1950.
12. MAKOUS N, FRIEDMAN S, YAKOVAC W and MARIS EP. Cardiovascular manifestations in progeria. Report of clinical and pathologic findings in a patient with severe arteriosclerotic heart disease and aortic stenosis. *Am Heart J* **64**: 334, 1962.
13. MORAN JJ and BECKER SM. Idiopathic arterial calcification of infancy: Report of 2 cases occurring in siblings, and review of the literature. *Am J Clin Pathol* **31**: 517, 1959.
14. MOVITER ER, GERSTL B, SHERWOOD F and EPSTEIN CC. Essential hypertension. *Arch Intern Med* **87**: 79, 1951.
15. NEUFELD HN, LESTER RG, ADAMS P JR, ANDERSON RC, LILLEHEI CW and EDWARDS JE. Congenital communication of a coronary artery with a cardiac

chamber or the pulmonary trunk ("coronary artery fistula"). *Circulation* **24**: 171, 1961.

16. NEUFELD HN, WAGENVOORT CA, ONGLEY PA and EDWARDS JE. Hypoplasia of ascending aorta. An unusual form of supravalvular aortic stenosis with special reference to localized coronary arterial hypertension. *Am J Cardiol* **10**: 746, 1962.

17. RAGHIB G, BLOEMENDAAL RD, KANJUH VI and EDWARDS JE. Aortic atresia and premature closure of foramen ovale. Myocardial sinusoids and coronary arteriovenous fistula serving as outflow channel. *Am Heart J* **70**: 476, 1965.

18. SCHAEFER LE, DRACHMAN SR, STEINBERG AG and ADLERSBERG D. Genetic studies on hypercholesteremia: Frequency in a hospital population and in families of hypercholesteremic index patients. *Am Heart J* **46**: 99, 1953.

19. SCHIMKE RN, MCKUSICK VA, HUANG T and POLLACK AD. Homocystinuria: Studies of 20 families with 38 affected members. *JAMA* **193**: 711, 1965.

20. STRAUSS L. The pathology of gargoylism: Report of a case and review of the literature. *Am J Pathol* **24**: 855, 1948.

21. TALBOT NB, BUTLER AM, PRATT EL, MACLACHLAN EA and TANNHEIMER J. Progeria: Clinical, metabolic and pathologic studies on a patient. *Am J Dis Child* **69**: 267, 1945.

22. THOMAS WA, LEE KT, MCGAVRAN MH and RABIN ER. Endocardial fibroelastosis in infants associated with thrombosis and calcification of arteries and myocardial infarcts. *N Engl J Med* **255**: 468, 1956.

23. TRAISMAN HS, LIMPERIS NM and TRAISMAN AS. Myocardial infarction due to calcification of the arteries in an infant. *Am J Dis Child* **91**: 34, 1956.

24. VAN CREVELD S. Coronary calcification and thrombosis in an infant. *Ann Pediatr (Paris)* **157**: 84, 1941.

25. VLODAVER Z and NEUFELD HN. The coronary arteries in coarctation of the aorta. *Circulation* **37**: 449, 1968.

26. VLODAVER Z and EDWARDS JE. The coronary vessels in cases with pulmonary atresia and in cases with aortic atresia with intact ventricular septum (unpublished data).

27. WILKERSON CF, HAND EA and FLIGELMAN MT. Essential familial hypercholesterolemia. *Ann Intern Med* **29**: 671, 1948.

28. WILLIAMS RR, KENT GB JR and EDWARDS JE. Anomalous cardiac blood vessel communicating with the right ventricle: Observations in a case of pulmonary atresia with an intact ventricular septum. *Arch Pathol* **52**: 480, 1951.

A B 5
C 6
D 7
E 8
F 9
G 0
H 1
I 2
J 3